Lifting

THE BULL

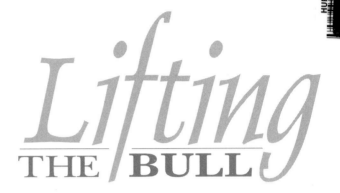

Best wishes
for better health,

D. Dawber

Other Books by Diane Dawber

Reading To Heal:
A Reading Group Strategy for Better Health

My Underwear's Inside Out:
The Care and Feeding of Young Poets

How Do You Wrestle a Goldfish?

Oatmeal Mittens

Cankerville

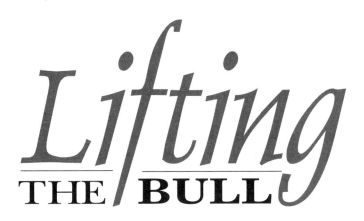

Lifting
THE BULL

Overcoming

Chronic Back Pain

Fibromyalgia
&
Environmental Illness

Diane Dawber

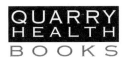

The publisher acknowledges The Canada Council for the Arts and the Book Publishing Industry Development Program of the Department of Canadian Heritage for supporting the arts of writing and publishing in Canada.

The publisher does not advocate the use of any particular treatment program, but believes that the information presented in this book should be available to the public. The nutritional, medical, and health information presented in this book is based on the research, training, and personal experiences of the author, and is true and complete to the best of the author's knowledge. However, this book is intended only as an informative guide for those wishing to know more about good health. It is not intended to replace or countermand the advice given by the reader's physician. Because there is always some risk involved, the author and publisher are not responsible for any adverse effects or consequences resulting from any of the suggestions made in this book. And because each person and each situation is unique, the author and the publisher urge the reader to consult with a qualified health professional before using any procedure where there is a question as to its appropriateness. It is a sign of wisdom, not cowardice, to seek a second or third opinion.

ISBN 1-55082-199-7

Design by Susan Hannah.
Typesetting and proofreading by Kate Archibald-Cross.

Back cover photograph by Michael Lea, courtesy of the Kingston *Whig Standard*.

Printed and bound in Canada by AGMV, Cap-St-Ignace, Quebec.

Published by Quarry Press Inc.,
P.O. Box 1061, Kingston, Ontario K7L 4Y5,
www.quarrypress.com

Contents

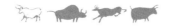

Steamed Open

I find

Virginia Woolf
in a room of her own
dining & smoking & drinking
followed
by a sudden altering of mood
attributed to a tailless cat
& drowning herself like an unwanted kitten;

Sylvia Plath
in her bell jar
and a bout of food poisoning
requiring mental hospitalization
throwing up her life
ironically with her head in an oven;

Edna, my mother
poet of the local papers
banging up her car
and then banging out her life
with the 'twenty-two';

& the critics admonish me
for my fixation on meaning
when there are language's sensory delights
available for their ears
which cannot hear
the screaming of bodies
my body
screaming

& I have steamed open
the message
hot hours in a fever
to avert the cold ending.

Foreword

I've always been good in a crisis, not falling apart until everything was over. In 1974, our basement flooded a foot deep, the furnace went off, and the outside temperature plunged from 0 degrees Fahrenheit to -18 degrees in several hours. I was the one who stayed home, called for pump rentals, furnace repair, and insurance adjusters. When my husband was in the hospital for six weeks in the fall of 1982, I taught full-time, looked after our two kids, went to the hospital every day, and tried to keep up with the Master's degree course (my first), which I had unfortunately started four days before.

Chronic illness shifted my ability to cope into a different register, however. I still managed to cope with outside crises, but what upset me most was my body. While learning to monitor every action for hazards to my back (not just too heavy a load but too far a reach, too fast a motion, or just a position held too long), I frequently came up against my limitations. The penalty for one wrong move was an uncontrollable chain reaction of pain that would last an indefinite length of time — hours if I was lucky, days or weeks if I wasn't.

That wasn't all. Each episode narrowed the limitations. My body was like an invisible electric fence in which I had become entangled, without an off-switch in reach. Each time I blundered, I felt an unfamiliar panic. The panic was

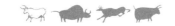

enough to make me feel even worse. If anyone chastised me for the panic, I felt all the more upset. I didn't want to feel this way or have others see me this way. I know they felt almost as helpless as I. For me, at least, there was the determination that I would get past this time and learn — learn not to blunder the same way twice. It was like mapping an invisible minefield by tapping around with a toe.

"Why not stay put?" you say.

To stay put was to stay in the cage. The only way out seemed to be to go as close to the limits as possible, without setting off the minefield. For some reason, that seemed to push the limitations outward, just a fraction. The next day, I could do one more repetition of an exercise, stay at an activity for a couple of minutes more, lift an ounce more, all the while alert for the danger of overuse.

Then there was the medical and health community to cope with, the psychotherapists, physiotherapists, the various specialists, and the even less well-informed and dispassionate.

"My attitude in this is that we treat the patient for depression first and then we can see what we've got."

"What if I had a broken leg?"

That point gets lost and remains unanswered by the locum.

"I've discussed this with my colleague and she agrees."

I didn't say anything. There's no point wasting energy talking to someone whose mind is made up. When the doctor doesn't know what is wrong, he or she can pass the buck to a specialist, and, failing that, blame the patient for imagining herself into this state. I'm sure there are many good therapists who help many people with many problems, but there aren't many who can figure out a wrecked back or cure an actual physical disease.

Pain is fatiguing. It takes mental effort to close it off from what you're doing. It takes mental effort to keep thinking about other things instead of the pain. Pain is like a small

child crying. Distraction can work for a while, but, if there is really something wrong, distraction eventually loses. I know quite a few people who have been sent to psychiatrists, psychologists, etc. for help with their fibromyalgia. Those who found someone who gave help with pain control strategies are fortunate. What we need is help to take back some control in our lives, not exhausting and exhaustive discussions of our childhoods or relationships. There is no energy for such luxuries. We're talking survival here.

The rehabilitation specialist took the long view.

"What you have is a total body syndrome," he said. "Intellectual, emotional, physical, and spiritual." He held up a piece of paper with a quartered circle drawn on it.

"What if a person breaks a leg?"

"Perhaps the person was rushing because she was emotionally upset because she was spiritually out of harmony."

"Hmm," I said, and thought that a piece of ice hidden by snow on the sidewalk was a more satisfactory explanation.

'Nothing is an accident,' is the philosophy of these people. It is more likely that a heck of a lot of things are accidents. You can trace a cause-and-effect relation only so far. Total body syndrome is pushing it a little too far, I think. However, it could be a short-circuiting of the cause-and-effect train by going to cosmic sorts of causes instead of trying to untangle the nearby ones. I have been guilty of that myself.

How can we tell when to look for causes and when to acknowledge the role of accident? What if, most of the time, we should be looking for physical causes and admitting defeat only when our know-how breaks down? Wild-goose chases after psychological causes may do more harm than good by making the person more helpless and dependent than ever.

To be fair, this was the same specialist who showed me a stretch which saves my bacon constantly. The iliapsoas release consists of lying down, pushing my hip toward my

feet with one hand while pulling my ribcage toward my head with the opposite hand. This simple movement usually keeps my sciatica from flaring up.

Then there was this gem from another physical specialist: "Fibromyalgia patients tend to do what's comfortable in exercise, not what's right."

I couldn't believe he said that! I don't want to believe he said that! It came out so easily and hits so hard. To be fair again, the statement can be interpreted two ways. One is that fibromyalgia patients are hedonistic cows, only interested in their own comfort. The other, more charitable, is that fibromyalgics avoid inflicting pain on themselves, even for "their own good."

I spent two years following exercise suggestions which sank me deeper and deeper into a downward spiral of pain and muscle spasms until I was virtually unable to move. Books like Hamilton Hall's *The Back Doctor* try to sort patients with back pain into four categories with appropriate exercises for each, and I know that for some people they do work, but he has only one page on fibromyalgia and it is not helpful. Perhaps because we do not 'fit' the categories, it assumes there is something the matter with us instead of something the matter with his system.

I spent another year gingerly trying out more suggestions like acupuncture, aquabics, Tai Chi, yoga — you name it, I tried it — which landed me in blinding pain over and over again. I spent more time painfully rebuilding my back muscles one miserable step at a time with little to guide me but the reactions of my own body. To say to me that I tend to do what's comfortable not only sounds ludicrous but feels cruel and spiteful to me.

Here are some examples of "doing what's comfortable": Asked to do "step-ups" by the sports injury specialist, I bent over, got one foot up and leaned on my knee to get the other up.

"No, no! Stand up straight. Hands at your sides."

I try to do it, not quite succeeding, and leaving my muscles shaking and knotting and burning for days. At home, I try a tiny stair step between my living and dining rooms; a year later, after doing this tiny step every day as many times as I can, I can do it standing straight. It wasn't a lack of desire but a lack of ability.

Asked to lie on my back with my arms at my sides and my palms facing the ceiling, I try, but my back, chest, and shoulder muscles immediately knot. It is useless to resist the pain and spasms which pull my hands over my chest, palms down. Two years later, I can practice the hands-at-side, palms-up position, and can often hold it for a whole minute.

"Breathe," says the yoga teacher, "from your abdomen."

I am taking shallow breaths with my chest. My abdominal muscles are knotted; my back muscles are knotted. Even the tiny movements of a shallow chest breath hurt. Three years later, I can breathe almost normally.

"Just lie on your front on the bench," says the physiotherapist. Soon after, he puts in the acupuncture needles which will help rid me of a bad headache. After he leaves, I find it hard to breathe. My right shoulder, arm, and hand begin to tighten and then to shake with spasms. I try to relax it but the pain blanks out thought. I wish I could pass out. Later adjustments — like lying on pillows, a rolled towel to angle my neck in an easier position, a bench with drop-down arm rests, a heat pack under my chest during the treatment — all make it possible to have the acupuncture with fewer problems.

Is this what is meant by "doing what's comfortable?" It seems to me that the visible signs should indicate to the professionals that there is a physical problem somewhere that is not being addressed. After they were addressed by myself or someone else, things started to improve. I could do what was required "properly" because I was able.

Foreword

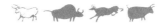

Perhaps the problem here was that it is almost impossible for a person not so afflicted to imagine the pain. If I try to describe it, that may help.

There is a kind of pain in which you cannot keep still. Imagine trying to keep still with your hand slammed in a door. Somehow the frantic movement distracts the brain from the alarm signals shooting up the arm. I had many days when I was totally exhausted but simply could not stop my restless motion because if I did, the pain flooded up my spine until it pulsed head to toe. Somehow, just keeping moving blocked the sensation a bit. But moving just exacerbated the resulting deluge of pain. I froze part of myself with ice packs, seven at times, rotating them from pain point to pain point.

There is another kind of pain that makes any normal activity an exercise in agony. Imagine waking in the morning with a stiff neck, such a stiff neck that it hurts even to turn your eyes left and right, so stiff that you can't move to get out of bed. Begin with a tiny rocking motion, and half an hour later it is free enough so you can roll over and get up. Imagine you're taking a shower and you want to shampoo your hair. However, your shoulder is so stiff you cannot raise your arm to do it. You stand with the heat and water beating down on your right shoulder. When it's practically scalded numb, you kneel on the bottom of the tub and prop your arm on the tub edge for support as you try to shampoo. Now try to get out of the tub without using your arms much or bending your back much. Don't slip or move suddenly because the pain hits so hard it takes your breath away.

Put your clothes on with the same problems.

Breakfast? Try to reach a plate on the first shelf. Try to lift the juice jug or the kettle.

Tired of the pain yet? How many hours to go until bed-time?

Wait! I haven't got a headache yet. Remember, I have a

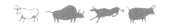

stiff neck. I want to wash my plate and glass but try to do it without looking down. I bring my cup of tea to the table and open the newspaper. In fifteen minutes, or less, my neck, scalp, eyelids have gone into spasms. This is what the doctor calls a "tension headache."

Now I'll have to lie down, listen to the radio, try to rest, try not to stay in one position long enough to stiffen there. TV is out because I can't lie or sit in position long enough. Books and magazines are a problem for the same reason.

Standing up is the best alternative to lying down, so I go for a walk. Trouble is I need smooth, fairly level ground, so I have to drive to a local park or to the mall in winter. But driving is excruciating because of the stiff neck, pain on raising the arms, and pain on pressing the accelerator or brake.

Half an hour for a walk. Be careful not to stumble on a root or stone or slip in a bit of mud. It's hard when you can't look down very well, but the penalty for a slip is a painful jarring of the head, neck, and back. The least uphill bit strains the lower back. Looking up at a squirrel or woodpecker strains the neck and back. I wear a jacket with pockets at chest level that ease the weight of my arms. The mall isn't much easier, with its hard floors and many temptations to look sideways or down. Birthday cards and books are the worst, requiring a sideways look which promptly brings on another headache.

But what about medication? Surely a few painkillers would help the discomfort. I've tried them all. Eight ASA tablets a day added ringing ears to the problems. Acetaminophen and ibuprofen don't help much either. Besides that, many pills make the mind as groggy and foggy as a humid night in July.

As a writer and teacher, I found the interference with my mind the most terrifying of all. Already the bedtime medication — 50 mg of amitriptyline — had caused some fogginess and a loss of some processes, such as metaphoric thinking. I

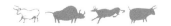

relieved it a little by taking the medication in the early evening instead of at bedtime. Painkillers on top of this made for a pretty sad brain as well.

And there is another kind of pain that is so bad you must keep still. It hurt so much to breathe at times I could only take little sips of air. I couldn't move any part of myself — my head, my arms, my legs, my torso, my very eyelids — without stabbing pain everywhere. The only way I survived those days and nights was to lie very still and use a Zen strategy of counting my breaths up to ten and then starting over. My mind could not handle anything more or less. The human being shrinks to a point of breath. I shrank to a point of breath.

Through all this, you would think that my mind would have been on the back problem. That would have been much too logical. No, I was worried that my back problem was the result of some kind of character or personality defect. This psychological guilt, this spiritual malaise, was another kind of pain. Now why would a person who had survived her mother's suicide, her father's devastation by rheumatoid arthritis, her husband's bankruptcy and illness — and twenty-five years of simultaneous teaching, studying for two degrees, writing two books, child-rearing, and household management — think that she lacked fiber? Constipation? And what makes it worse is that the medical profession is eager to let us blame ourselves, because it beats trying to figure out what is wrong with that delicate instrument, the back — or with society's demands on it.

In her Booker Prize winning novel, *The Ghost Road*, Pat Barker refers to soldiers from the First World War writing journals, letters, diaries, poems, etc. in a desperate attempt to avert death. If you are in the midst of writing something,

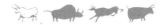

then surely you will stay alive to finish it. In books, the narrator usually survives to tell the tale. And the writer cheats death of some of its power to obliterate the person.

Perhaps that's why I began writing this book while feeling that desperation, that fear of obliteration. Surely, if I started writing, then I would figure out my problem and recover. At the worst of times, feeling like giving up, an inner voice would say, "That won't make a very good book. No one wants to read about a failure." A very slender thread on which to hang a life but maybe no more slender than many others.

Although some health care professionals told me that what I was suffering was "not life-threatening," they were wrong. I could have died, probably of a stroke. Aside from that, the unrelenting pain might have eventually driven me to suicide. I was right to be afraid. I was right to keep looking for answers. I was right to reject what didn't contribute to progress. My only shame is that I knew so little about protecting my own health and the health of my family at home and my students at school. I knew so little about what has been happening to our environment and our food.

This may sound a bit dramatic, over the top — unless, of course, you are there too, in pain. To survive took so much effort that I want to share my strategies with you in hope of easing your passage to better health. I was lucky that my condition was so severe because it was an impetus to improve or die in the attempt. I was lucky I have my father's determination and the desire to learn how to heal myself. I had the good fortune to become ill just as there was an explosion of knowledge about alternative healing strategies. I had the education to help me read books and articles about my illness. I had the financial resources (thanks to private and public health insurance plans) to pursue answers. And I had my creative streak to give me metaphors to use in exploring. The metaphor of "Lifting the Bull" came to me as I read a small folktale :

There was once a farmer who gave his son a calf. "Son," he said, "lift this calf every day. As it slowly grows bigger, your muscles will become stronger and stronger. By the time you and the calf grow up, you will be able to lift a whole bull."

After five years of being bested by the bull of pain, I slowly built strength to lift the beast and even throw it. I also learned the difference between that other kind of bull and the truth.

So here is my story — stupidities, despair, struggles, and triumphs — warts and all.

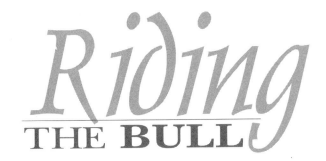

Riding
THE BULL

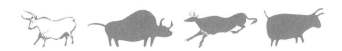

Holding Up My End

Good health. For years I had experienced what I believed was good health with only a few minor problems — ailments like the common cold and a small neuroma on my foot — all treatable by physicians, surgeons, and pharmaceuticals supplied to care for me by public and private health care plans. I took this state of affairs for granted until a wee beastie started a chain reaction that radically changed my understanding of the meaning of good health, medicine, and myself.

When you are busy swatting a gnat, you don't notice the steam roller bearing down. I was busy swatting a gnat — or, in this case, a head louse — when the steam roller hit.

11/88 It began with a case of head lice, or rather the twenty-fifth case of head lice, mine. Most schools have a small percentage of children with head lice. That year, the school where I was teaching ended up with an unusually high number of chronic cases. Too many to dilute. Almost all our students rode school buses, which made for a lot of shoulder to shoulder contact. A head lice paradise!

The head lice population exploded. At one point, seventy per cent of the students and staff were afflicted, picking nits and shampooing with prescribed mixtures. Teachers were

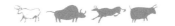

not immune. Three or four had already gone through the routine. It was one time we envied our principal's growing baldness.

I was teaching at a country school with about 200 children, kindergarten to grade 8. It was a school where "if you close your eyes real tight, you see cow pats and not spots," as Canadian poet Al Purdy would put it. I prefer cow pats to city traffic so that was no problem to me. It was a pleasant little school, albeit a bit crowded, with the library in a portable and the staff room in a nine-by-nine kitchen.

That year was our first to offer junior kindergarten and we had a bumper crop — so many that we had to divide them into two classes. Junior kindergarten was scheduled for alternate days. The principal looked over the staff for a suitable teacher. I was alternating the role of school librarian and Grade 5-6 teacher. I seemed like a logical choice, from his perspective.

From my own, it seemed a lot less logical and a lot more like the easy way out. I was, and am, very interested in the teaching of writing and had myself written two books. Not much chance for writing in Junior Kindergarten, I thought.

I hadn't taught a primary grade for fifteen years, except for the assistance I rendered as librarian to our primary classes. My last experience teaching primary had been thirty-nine grade two students in another school and under a different system. It had not been a particularly enjoyable year. Junior kindergarten didn't seem appealing.

My back had been giving me trouble off and on for years, including a four-year stint limping with an undiagnosed Morton's neuroma, a foot tumor which teachers often get from standing so much, consisting of nerve tissue between two metatarsal joints. It was eventually discovered and removed, but left me with problems on the left side from the limping. Without having it identified as such, I had a chronic pain problem then, but the worst of it had been relieved by

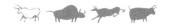

surgery to remove the neuroma. A small car accident four years before hadn't helped either. Often enough, I had pain down my left side from neck to toes. So far, it was ignorable and treatable with painkillers and rest. No — junior kindergarten with all that bending didn't seem appealing at all.

Despite the fact that there was little or nothing in the way of equipment for a second junior kindergarten room, I scrounged at home and yard sales. My room was ready by September. Then I was told that the numbers of older children required a re-shuffling of rooms and my re-setting up in two-thirds of a classroom formerly used for special education. This was going to be special, too.

The children themselves, though not ready to take creative writing classes, soon showed they could provide mountains of material for one. One tiny fellow (who arrived with his mom in matching jean jackets decorated with Twisted Sister stickers) gave a lot all by himself. His angelic wouldn't-say-boo-to-a-goose table mate turned liquid blue eyes to me at one of the first lunch times and whispered in distress, "Ms Dawber, I've got a sandwich on my neck!" And so he did, applied by his neighbor who was hooting with laughter. The other children were not quite sure whether to be impressed or appalled. The tiniest girl, in patent shoes and ruffles sniffed, "That's what boys do. Girls don't do that." And I could see the sturdy tomboy beside her ready to disagree. As I say, it was interesting material and I was beginning to enjoy myself.

So here I was, helping my fourteen junior kindergartners with their hats and coats and mittens and scarves when the head lice epidemic struck. The numbers in every class ebbed and flowed as new cases and even repeat cases occurred. For two weeks, I was lucky. The frequent "head check," carried out by volunteer parents and anyone else we could dragoon, had, so far, given me a clean bill of health.

The classroom was made as safe as possible, with stuffed

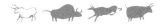

animals and dress-up clothes sealed in plastic bags for the duration. The other teachers and I conducted some of the head checks ourselves as volunteers wore out. The discovery of new cases was always upsetting for the children, their parents, the rest of the class, and the teachers. I reassured distraught parents that clean scalps were no deterrent — in fact, what bug wouldn't prefer pleasant quarters. The grim lines of their mouths did not relax much. Some became exhausted, desperate and angry after two or more episodes of buying the expensive shampoo. Not to mention that all this was after spending all their spare time checking their children's and their own heads and washing, vacuuming, and wiping down everything in their houses. The dry-cleaning bills were not insignificant either. Everyone's emotions were strained from dealing with upset children and upset adults.

One night, I stopped by the local hospital to visit a parent who had done volunteer work for me. I dropped off a few flowers, gave her a hug, and was on my way with an unsuspected passenger. Hospitals are not amused if they find out you have head lice, so the patient was afraid to say anything until she got out and back home. She was one who had been through the routine twice with two daughters whose blond hair made it difficult to see the little beasts.

The nits sure showed up a couple of days later in my dark mop, perhaps already dead because I had, on no more evidence than an itchy scalp (which we all imagined all the time), already used the medicated shampoo. Anyway, I went home, in a state of fatigue and upset, to a disbelieving male chorus at home.

"Don't you think you're overreacting, Hon?" said the senior male, Chris, when I asked for help with the vacuuming.

"What a pain! I've got a group coming over to watch the election results! We'll have to go somewhere else," said my politically-active older son, Michael, when I mentioned that everything would have to be laundered.

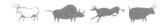

"You're making too much of this, Mum," said my younger son, Matthew, when I announced that coats would have to go the cleaners or be sealed up in plastic bags.

Before I did anything else, though, I had to check through three mercifully dark heads of hair.

"There better not be anything there," said Chris. And there wasn't, though I teased that gray hairs made it tricky to tell.

"If there is anything in my hair, I'm going to kill!" said Mike. And, luckily for the penal system, there wasn't.

"Hurry up, Mom. I've got band practice in half an hour. This is really ridiculous," said Matthew. Unfortunately it was pediculous not ridiculous.

"I guess you got it because we both like the sofa by the TV. It's okay. Just use the shampoo and I'll check for a few days. Dad, you're going to have to check me for a few days, too."

"Jeez," he said shuddering. "I don't even know what the buggers look like. Can't you get someone else?"

"Well, here's the nit I just took out of number two son's hair. It looks just like a piece of dandruff down near the roots, but it sticks to the hair while a piece of dandruff slides off easily."

"I guess," and he plunged his head back into the newspaper.

I took out my frustration on the house. I took the bedding off all the beds and started it through the wash. I vacuumed each room as carefully as I could, along the baseboards, behind everything, in the closets and even up the curtains. I bagged the clothes in my closet and in Matt's. I bagged extra coats in the closets and took the ones being worn to the cleaners. I vacuumed the furniture, especially that favorite spot on the sofa by the TV. Cleaning up took me long into the evening and, by the time I was tucking new sheets and blankets under the mattresses, I was finding it hard to bend. I was pretty stiff. I was pretty mad at the lack of assistance, too. I had

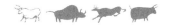

considered calling my cleaning lady, but I wasn't sure she'd even step a foot inside our house again if she found out we had head lice. No sense calling a cleaning company in the middle of the evening. Would they even be able or willing to fit me in on short notice? I guess that's why I took the line of least resistance and did it myself.

The next morning I was stiff, especially in the left shoulder blade area and left hip. There was still a pile of blankets to launder, and I had to do a head check on everyone, so I called the school and told them not to expect me. The day after that, I went back, satisfied that everything had been deloused, even if the help had been lousy and I was feeling lousier still.

It was junior kindergarten day and, as usual, the children coming from the bus would arrive at the classroom door, deposit their lunches, show-and-tell impedimenta, library books and other gear, go to the washroom assisted by a bigger buddy (lots of these children had been on the bus for over half an hour) and then go on out to play. The other junior kindergarten teacher and I had decided that, rather than endure another donning and removal of snowsuits at recess, we would have a longer playtime outdoors right after the buses arrived. These children had been sitting for long enough and needed a chance to wear off a build-up of suppressed kinetic energy.

They always bounce out the door like watch-springs released from cases. Since it was just cold with not much snow, the tricycles and the wagon went too. I followed to supervise the swinging, the climbing, and the disputing over the tricycle. One particularly tall and athletic girl, used to competing with brothers, was liable to decide that the tricycle was there for her undivided use. Separating her from it, if she disagreed, was like detaching a starving octopus from a lucky catch.

That day was mostly calm, and I resisted any pleas for little pushes on the swings because my back was still sore. We began

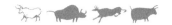

the last round-up to send the children, far-flung on the school yard, in to begin Show and Tell. The last two were galloping in, pulling a third child in our big wooden wagon, when the handle and two front wheels detached from the rest, sending the three into orbit. Checking that they were unhurt, I sent them in and tried to juggle the pieces together, but I ended up carrying the lot — a heavy lot — which made my back feel even worse. Why did I do it myself and not send someone else? As usual, it was quicker than trying to look after my class while trying to find someone and explain the problem. Again, the line of least resistance.

By the end of the day, I was bushed, but reasoned that the next day — a professional development day for planning the next term and attending a school meeting about the head lice problem — would rest my back.

The school library, for which I was responsible, had a number of tables, some rectangular, which I easily and regularly repositioned for different activities. The table which we were going to use for the staff potluck looked just like the tables in the library, gray with a laminate top. I lifted my end and something told me that this table was much bigger and heavier than the ones I normally used. What told me was a sickening "give" in the middle of my spine. Since I was sore already, it didn't seem much different, just more so. Why didn't I leave the job to someone else? Just trying to "hold up my end," I guess.

That's all that happened really. I went to the doctor and came away with advice to take painkillers, put on ice, and rest up, which I did for the weekend.

Every day at school after that, when I went to bend, my back didn't want to bend. It did anyway — bent to help a child with a persnickety mitten, bent to help a child with a snarly zipper, bent to help a child with a Gordian knot for a shoelace, bent to help a child with a booby-trapped pudding cup or thermos lid tightened by Hercules, bent to look at a child's

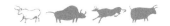

block construction or painting or coloring or beadwork, bent to examine a bumped finger or skinned knee or pouting lip. Every bend required more effort to overcome my back's reluctance to do so. It wasn't so much pain as it was a stiffness. If it had been an excruciating pain, perhaps I would have gone for attention sooner. I have since found out that we are not able to identify pain in that region as readily because our brains have fewer correlating pain receptors.

01/89 Back to the doctor I went and came out with the second line of attack — anti-inflammatories. In with the anti-inflammatories and off to outer space. I was floating in a mental rubber-dinghy on a plume of forgetfulness high above the junior kindergarten. I could see my students far below. It was just that much farther to bend.

After a few days, the rubber raft descended a notch, but I began to feel nauseated. Perhaps all that floating was making me seasick. That didn't help at all, so I forgot the anti-inflammatories. Just too much aggravation for no relief.

02/89 "You mean you quit taking the pills?" said the doctor.

"Well, they made me feel sick to my stomach and didn't seem to be helping. It's hard enough to teach with a sore back without feeling as if I'm going to throw up any minute."

Doctors do not like it when you stop taking their pills without immediate notice. However that may be, I was put on a list for physiotherapy. At this point, I still believed (and the doctor obviously believed) that this pain was going to go away like the ninety-nine per cent of pains that people have. The fact that this had been going on for several months should have been a warning flag. Any pain that lasts that long is chronic already, by definition.

Physiotherapy

One day, I arrived at my classroom and perched on the edge of a junior-kindergarten-sized table. I did that because I felt I couldn't sit down even if I had a normal chair. I couldn't bend my head at all. I paged the principal. The superintendent, who had helped persuade me to take junior kindergarten, happened to be there too.

"What's the matter, Di?"

"I'm going to have to go back home."

"What's the matter?"

"I can't bend."

"Why not?"

"I'm not sure. My back hurts."

"Oh."

03/89 There is no record for that day in my journal or for several days after that. I went home and called the doctor, and the doctor called the physiotherapist to take me right away. It was almost March school break anyway, so I stayed home a couple of days and rested.

The first encounter with physiotherapy was for assessment. Almost everything I was asked to do, I couldn't or

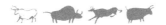

could do only with difficulty. Bending forward was the worst. It took hands on the walls and assistance to get back up. There I was wailing about my stresses of yore while hand-over-handing-it up the wall to stand straight again after bending. If ever a person needed to be told not to be so daft, I was that person. Unfortunately, no one did. However, the physiotherapist did know me slightly as a teacher, so I was not discounted as an hysteric immediately.

By Easter Monday, I knew I was in trouble. When I tried to bend my head enough to look at the phone book — which was on the dining room table to look up the number for a substitute teacher — not only was it tough to do, but my head erupted in a furious headache.

The doctor sent me home for a month of rest on 100 mg of amitriptyline. Nothing wrong with that you say? Taking the stuff was like substituting pink insulation for brain cells. My usual mental functioning was altered with little explanation or reassurance. Since I assumed the medication was temporary, I lay down and tried to cope with the pain and the fog and the exercises recommended.

Since I was having trouble bending, the exercises tried to address that. Curling up in a knee hug was one. Hooking my hands behind my knees and pulling my leg up was another. My whole body hurt with each repetition.

After a month, I went back to the medical people and was assured that, even though I hurt, it was fine to go back to work. Fine if I was a crash-test dummy or a bed-tester, was my opinion, especially since I was supposed to keep on taking the brain-fuzzifying medication. Lots of people take much more of the stuff in its anti-depressant application. How depressing for them if they have to exchange their anxieties for this.

Chris didn't think I was ready to go back. My step-mom didn't think I was ready to go back. I didn't think I was ready either, but the combination of medical reassurance and guilt

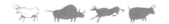

over upsetting my class of tiny tots by deserting them in their first year of school made me go back. The theory is that most pain goes away. Most times it does.

At my next physiotherapy appointment, the x-rays showed a sacrilization — a bony attachment to the third lumbar vertebra. It can cause problems with the functioning of the back, especially with bending. The physiotherapist advised me to give up the idea of teaching kindergarten.

That was at two o'clock and at four o'clock the school board held its teacher transfer meeting. I thought it was my only chance to change my assignment from kindergarten. I roared in, chose a grade 2-3 at another school, and roared out. My principal gave me the dickens for not warning him. I would have liked more warning, too.

"We could have worked something else out," he said.

It was about this time that I went to see a specialist. He suggested a TENS® unit, which I could wear to work to alleviate the pain. I had been having some TENS® treatments at physiotherapy and it seemed to help a little. The theory was that the pain was causing the spasms which caused more pain and so on. That seemed reasonable. The TENS® unit sends a minute electrical current across the skin between the electrodes and the electrical current interferes with the pain signal. So I wore the thing, two electrodes at the top of my back and two at the bottom. The sensation was a small buzz, which wasn't bothersome. The wires leading to the battery pack and controls made some motions awkward, which was all to the good, because those motions didn't make my back any better. As I now know, there is a problem. The nervous system learns the pattern and then ignores it. Why couldn't it just ignore the pain pattern instead?

Every morning, Chris had to tape the electrodes to my back and every evening, remove them. I had to wear skirts and blouses that would allow the cords to pass through to the black box that I wore on my waistband. The children at

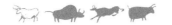

school, of course, were curious and I tried to explain. I'm sure some thought I had a magical device to record their behavior, communicate with the principal or administer rude shocks to miscreants.

Unfortunately, the TENS® unit and the theory pushed me to ignore the pain. That turned out to be the wrong thing to do. I just kept going, increasing fatigue, increasing adrenaline to fight the pain *and* the fatigue — and thereby increasing the pain in a vicious circle. The more pain was ignored, the more muscles went into spasms and weakened.

Things got worse, soon.

Yoga

All summer, I walked every day, two kilometers mostly, and tried to rest. It was rest, if you consider that grocery shopping, cooking, and so on with three men in the house can be classified as rest. Scheduling the car with two new drivers in the family car pool seemed like a full-time job, too. Worrying while they had the car was only moonlighting. Whoever said that it is so nice when children no longer needed their parents twenty-four hours a day was probably, but incorrectly, speaking about babyhood.

Another task was to introduce Michael to paid employment, which took a combination of goading, describing the delights of one's own money, and dragging him down to the office temp company. After passing all their tests with flying colors, he was soon doing their worst assignments with ease for the remainder of the summer — which was only August since it had taken me all of July to get him there.

I didn't rest easy on the medication either. I tried to reduce the amount, only to awaken in the night with terrible muscle cramps and accompanying anxiety. The doctor tried giving me a tranquilizer. I disliked the idea intensely but tried one. That night, I awoke again with the muscle cramps, with the only difference that I was perfectly calm while my body seized up.

08/89 I spent August putting together the going-off-to-university-for-the-first-time kit, which included such mundane things as a mending kit, a tool box, a flashlight and batteries, stationery supplies, first aid kit, snack kit, phone card, credit card, list of family birthdays (with mine prominently marked), laundry kit, and all the other impedimenta required by a child leaving home for eight months. I have the list still.

There is a picture of us on the day we drove Michael to Ottawa with his gear. I am in my horticultural battle dress, which allows me to fade into any flower bed with no one the wiser and which is exactly what I felt up to doing. Michael has a large grin. His dad is goofing around with sneakers on his ears to disguise his mixed feelings about Michael leaving home.

That fall I was teaching in a different school. That doesn't seem like much but it is equivalent to infiltrating enemy territory and sneaking into a well-defended munitions factory to steal their latest secret weapon. The kids don't know you and want to find out about you in the only way they know how. Since questions with no coercion are liable to elicit false answers, they torture. The Geneva Convention should spell out that one child asking to go to the washroom at every inconceivable inconvenient moment — as in when you are just going to explain the crux of the mathematics problems for that week — is enough. Every child in the class does not have to test your tolerance for interruptions. Likewise in the school yard, one child wading into every puddle every time you turn your back is quite enough.

The teachers aren't much better. They look into your classroom with a slight "tsk" if there are so many as two children speaking. They smile at your offers to plan cooperatively with pitying looks as if anyone in her right mind would want to be caught dead doing any of the ridiculous things your class does. The principal informs you that the cross-country

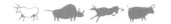

running team and rainy day recess duty in the gymnasium are all yours to enjoy. Your classroom is close to the boys' washroom, where the urinal plumbing has corroded and is leaking into the wall.

Actually, the class was adorable. I had met them the preceding June and looked forward to enjoying the activities I had planned for the year. Yet every day I was in pain. On many days I developed a raging headache. Some days I could barely move. It was a good thing the students were adorable and quite capable of doing whatever task I set them to do. They were quite accepting of the "black box" of the TENS® and the fact that I had a "bad back." They were a considerate group for eight-year-olds. I did the very best for them that I could.

On Mondays, Wednesdays, and often Fridays, I would get ready to go with the students at bus time, leave as soon as my darlings boarded, and drive like crazy to get to physiotherapy — a good half hour away by freeway. There was a black and white sign in the office warning that anyone missing an appointment would be charged (as in money or with a crime?) and that medicare would pay only part of the bill. The stern sign matched the expression of the receptionist.

The physiotherapist patiently tried every technique possible to get my snarled back to release the spasms. After TENS® came the Codatron®, a type of TENS®, with more electrodes which fire in a random pattern so that the nervous system cannot learn the pattern and then ignore it. Traction for the sciatica, manipulation, heat, cold, and a prescription of stretching exercises to be done every morning. Each day that I would arrive, face strained with pain, was another defeat, but neither of us considered giving up.

It was fortunate that the physiotherapist knew me slightly as a teacher at his children's school and had heard me address the school at the grade 8 graduation. I had some credibility. Otherwise, the miserable wreck, frightened and desperate,

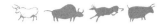

who appeared in his treatment room might have been dismissed as just another 'neurotic woman.' As it was, he took me seriously and was dismayed by my rapid deterioration.

On Mondays, after leaving from home at 7:30 a.m. for school, from school at 3:30 p.m. for physiotherapy, and from there at 4:30 for yoga classes, I would buy juice and sit in the car, drinking it and eating an apple. We weren't supposed to eat anything substantial before yoga class. Yoga was another strategy suggested by the specialist, so here I was, eager to get well and glad to have an excuse to exercise my curiosity, if nothing else.

Incense makes me choke. Ditto a place where people feel the need of it. Holiness has no smell for me unless it is plain, unvarnished fresh air. You can judge my mulishness right from the start. Perhaps I was mistaking a quest for holy smell for an attempt to cover up basement damp. Our lessons were in a basement room, nicely carpeted and painted white. We assembled in oddly-assorted bodies — it was a class for those with bad backs — and in oddly-assorted track suits, leotards, shorts, and what-have-you. Our leader, of course, was in white. Can't be a Devi in anything else.

We filled out information sheets and I had the usual irresistible urge to try and explain what the problem was. Since I didn't really know what to zero in on, my life story seemed a safe bet.

"Sit cross-legged on the end of your spine, soles of your feet together. Close your eyes. Breathe in and out from your abdomen. Focus your thoughts on your breath."

I was a minute into the first session and already I was in trouble. I couldn't sit on the end of my spine, couldn't put my feet together, couldn't close my eyes without spasms in the eyelids. It hurt to breathe at all, let alone from my abdomen, which was stiff as a board. I couldn't relax or focus on anything because of the overwhelming pain from everywhere. I managed to scoot back against a wall for support.

Yoga

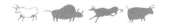

And then it got worse. If you have ever seen people or even pictures of people practicing yoga, you know that they get into "interesting" positions. Most of them require bending or raising some part of the anatomy, like arms or legs. Mine wouldn't raise — or, more accurately, they would raise along with the pain quotient. The final humiliation was lying on my back on the floor trying to turn my palms upward as instructed. Twisting my arms out of their sockets would have been just as comfortable.

The only part I enjoyed was lying down in darkness for a final relaxation. I felt I never wanted to do another thing except lie down in the dark, permanently, like some kind of human mushroom. When I got home, it was time for bed with a cozy complement of ice packs and pain pills. Nightmares about torture on the rack seemed inevitable.

Once, the instructor, trying to be helpful, suggested a massage. Now why did I think it would be any different from the classes? A subsequent Saturday morning found me lying naked on a table under a chilly sheet. I shivered with cold and fatigue, not a good beginning. When she dug her fingers into the hitherto-unsuspected tender spots on my chest, I squawked in a close approximation of a chicken having its feathers pulled — while alive. Tears ran down my face. It would be almost a year later that I would find out about the 'tender spots' of fibromyalgia.

"That's what's the matter with you. YOU'RE AFRAID. YOU'RE TERRIFIED!" she said.

Too right! I was too terrified to figure out that I was only afraid of her touching me again.

"This will help," she said as she dug her fingers into those spots again. "Just bear with it and it will be a lot better."

It wasn't. I babbled something about an unfortunate childhood and scurried into my clothes and out of there as quickly as I could.

You'd think that was enough — for any sensible person.

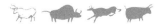

When you're so ill and have no inkling about why or how or anything, you keep trying to get better any way that offers. You've seen pictures of Hindu figures with many arms — well, this one got me with all of them. It took an actual further injury to sever me completely from the idea of yoga.

During that penultimate class in early 1990, we were lying on our fronts trying to push up into the cat or dog or hyena or whatever position it was. I was lying with my face into the mat with the yoga instructor encouraging me. I put my hands into position and pushed. Nothing. No strength in my arms or back.

"I can't," I said.

"Sure you can. Try! Come on!" she urged brightly.

"I can't."

"Just give a little push!"

Dammit! I gave a mighty heave, but just as I lurched up, something gave in my chest and I crashed to the mat in pain.

"Good for you! Are you all right?"

Too little. Too late. Or, rather, too much, too soon. It was home to ice and pills. Ice and pills for days. The pain in my chest reminded me of the pain that I had there a couple of years ago. That had lasted for at least two years. Someone less optimistic would have concluded a heart attack, and, I believe, some people, especially men, who get this pain are checked for heart attacks. It probably would have been a better option to go to Emergency and be put in bed for a couple of days as a possible heart attack.

Sternocostal chondritis (inflammation of the joint between the ribs and sternum) was the doctor's conclusion. At least it was a distraction from the back pain. At least it got me away from yoga for good.

This is not to say some positive things did not emerge from the experience. One night after class, in terrible pain, I called the instructor and she suggested a technique of focusing on the pain, visualizing it as a flame, in an effort to decrease the

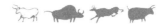

magnitude of the pain. I was to concentrate on the flame as it would get smaller and smaller and finally go out. Sometimes it does work for a while — a useful thing. Another technique is concentration on the breath. When other meditation or relaxation techniques fail because the pain is too great, concentration on the breath can allow me
 to get to sleep, though that is probably not the intended use.

There was another observation I made as I sat with the group being guided through a meditation. The instructor emphasized the heightened acuity of perception that would be ours. In fact, a dog barking, a car door slamming in the neighborhood, these already felt to me like a physical blow. My senses seemed to be turned up to an alarmingly sensitive pitch already. It was about this time that perfume became unbearable. The mildest scent of soap was too much. My skin reacted with prickling to anything but soft cotton. Perhaps I should have tried moving towards less perception.

In the same period that I was going to yoga classes, I was also swimming three times a week at the local Recreation Center. Swimming is recommended as the perfect exercise — warm, non-weight-bearing, relaxing, and so on. Let's deal with this mythology one point at a time. First of all, the warmth. In order to get into the warm pool, one has to take off one's clothes and put on a bathing suit in a chilly change room. If you don't have goose bumps yet, try the recommended pre-swim shower. Heads it's cool; tails it's cold. If you are really lucky, it's warm and even lasts awhile. Then you get to go out and shiver at poolside for the lifeguards to signal the all-clear. It seems to be making a lot out of minor annoyances, but the cold caused my muscles to tense and then to go into spasm. If you have pain localized in your finger, that may not be too bad. When you have it in your back or generalized to your whole body, muscles spasms can mean disabling headaches and days of misery.

In the evening — which was the only week-day time I had

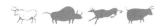

— our local pool has one lane roped off for laps. The rest is given over to children and a sprinkling of adults, all with different activities in mind, from water-sliding to playing with water polo balls. On good evenings, the other lap swimmers would come later, leaving me to paddle along slowly in the roped-off lane. Sooner or later, the lap-swimmers would be upon me, literally. One older, well-goggled fellow swam with the monotonous inflexibility of Jaws. I would try to duck out of the way or push myself quickly to the end to avoid those flailing arms. Others were good at passing me without hitting me, but their wake would wash over me unexpectedly, leaving me choking and snorting. When the adult lane became intolerable — that is, when I was half-drowned and tense as a springboard — I would duck under the rope and take my chances in the general area.

Breast stroke was about the only way to keep an eye out for the polo balls, flutter boards, or games of tag. Unfortunately, my neck would soon tire. The side or back stroke would give my neck a rest, but then I would have to contend with bumps, tidal waves, and kicks. If only I had learned to do the crawl when I was a youngster, but swimming lessons were not a part of life in those days.

One Saturday, cautiously side-stroking with a weather-eye out for an unusually large crowd, I noticed a swimmer in the roped lane. He was undoubtedly the pain specialist I had seen a few weeks before who had pressed various painful spots on my back and decided that since there was not an immediate reaction, there was nothing he could do for me. If there had been, it would have meant a chemical cocktail injected into the trigger points. I figured that the stress of getting to yet another appointment, waiting for the specialist, and taking off my clothes for another strange male already had my back in such a lock-up that dynamite would be needed to get a reaction.

He had diagnosed my condition as a chronic strain of

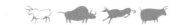

the trapezius, which left me not much the wiser. (Today I read that Repetitive Strain Injury is often described as a chronic strain of the trapezius.) He opined that, since there was no one obvious trigger point, he couldn't use the injection strategy.

After I had dressed, left his office, and got a mile down the road on that cold, dark February late afternoon, a spasm twisted the muscles of my mid-back so hard I considered pulling over. If I did, the knot would probably still not go away and I would be that much colder, more tired, and just as far away from home. Might as well carry on, so I did. It was probably the tiny bit of relaxation on heading for home that did it. There was room for the spasm to get a new grip.

"You'll strain yourself unless you swim properly with your head down," he said, heading out of the pool just as I reached the end. "Got to keep your head parallel with the water."

"Right," I thought, "and be a bumper boat!" I'd like to see him swim with his head down through the mess I was navigating. So much for relaxing.

Then it was time to get out, shiver into the shower, into the dressing room, into a cold, dark car, and home. My memories of this time are inordinately filled with the dark, the cold, and the inside of my car. Falling into bed was the only possible sequel but sleep was not the knitting of raveled sleeves of care. Well, just possibly, my past knitting results approached my sleep in raggedness.

Mondays I didn't get home from physiotherapy and yoga until around 9:30 p.m. Tuesdays and Thursdays I usually worked until 4:30 to make up for the days I had to leave school early (and even then, I had to take home a load of books to mark and preparation to do) and so reached home about five. Wednesdays and Thursdays I would go to physiotherapy and get home after five. Unfortunately, we were used to having dinner on the table at five because my husband's family was used to eating at five. I didn't care, although I'd

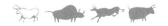

been used to dinner at six, because I could get all that out of the way early and have some evening before going to bed at 8:30.

Now, I wasn't home early enough to keep up the time-table so something had to give. Either we ate later or some-one else had to cook. Chris likes to cook. Anyone who didn't have to prepare dinner in twenty minutes 365 nights a year would like to cook. Pardon me. I exaggerate. Fifty-two nights a year we have pizza and we go out to a restaurant for our anniversary and a few other occasions. So, Chris took on more of the cooking. Michael, ditto. It wasn't just the cook-ing but the shopping and clearing up too. Most nights I was too whacked to do much of anything except the essentials for work the next day.

In May a strange thing began to happen. My husband's back began to act up. It was almost as if the extra load was the camel's straw for him, too. Then one day he went to pull up his trousers and it went. He had a couple of episodes over the years, ever since he had been switched from a desk job to loading boxcars during a strike. A heavy box lifted just the wrong way had done the damage. Every once in a while it reminded him. A few muscle relaxants, some ice, some heat, and he was fine.

I had a field trip organized for my class and another teacher's class as part of a water unit. Part of it was iffy — a visit to the Coast Guard Search and Rescue Station. They couldn't tell if an emergency would call them out, so I had an alternate plan ready. I was to call just before we were ready to leave the school and decide then which plan to use. Then Chris woke up unable to get out of bed, unable to even move without severe pain and muscle spasm — without a certain amount of choice language, too. Two hundred pounds of irate immobility.

I called the doctor and got his answering service.I called for a supply teacher. I called the doctor back. I called the supply teacher to explain the day's plans. I called the Coast

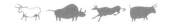

Guard, not to rescue me but to find out their status. I called the school to report the Coast Guard's availability. I called the doctor.

It sounds so easy now. By then it was nine a.m. and I had also boiled a hot pack, eaten something, got dressed, and fussed a lot. I called my husband's office to say he wouldn't be in.

The doctor came at ten. I went and got the prescription filled. I drove into the nearby city of Kingston, a good hour's trip, to get a commode. His office called back needing some information. I got some groceries; we still had to eat. Then a rest for an hour, reading.

For some reason, I made a batch of muffins. Why do I resort to cooking in a crisis? Perhaps it is familiar. Perhaps I have absorbed some chicken-soup theory of life somewhere. The best times I had as a kid were the ones helping my aunt make things like pies and fondant. When I got ready to be away from my kids for the first time, I made them a freezer full of cookies. Perhaps the way to remembrance is lined with baked goods.

I called the school to find out if the field trip had gone all right. Nobody knew. Eventually the supply teacher called to say everything had gone off just fine.

But my back didn't hurt. I had so much adrenaline running in my veins that I could have had an amputation without noticing.

Adrenaline is great in the crisis. It gets the brain moving faster ... and faster ... and ... you get the picture. What do you do with the leftovers — the leftover adrenaline? Package it up neatly and return to sender? Some people pray. Some people meditate. I didn't know anything about meditation except that Chris had tried it years ago. It was a washout for him because a neurological condition caused him to fall asleep at the wave of a mantra. My answer had always been to go out and mow the grass or wash windows or clean a

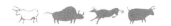

closet. Now I couldn't do that. Here I was with muscles already stiff and sore and with a pile of adrenaline that was making them tense up even more. Just coping with all my treatments and my regular schedule was enough.

Every day after that was a challenge and so the adrenaline just kept on flowing — until school let out for the summer. Then the reaction set in.

When I began writing this, I had an image in mind, an image of a caryatid, a pillar carved in the shape of a woman. Men, of course, can be Atlas, but women just get to be a nameless load-bearing column. In my case, as I tried to relax, I just got more and more tired. In the caryatid image, the carved column is transparent with the flesh-and-blood woman slumped in the bottom.

I didn't realize what was happening. I thought that the drug amitriptyline was making me groggy, so I tried to cut it back, which didn't help a bit. It seems stupid in retrospect. It only makes sense if you know how medication/disease/exhaustion affects the mental processes. I would try to take less amitriptyline so that I would be sharper mentally.

Halfway through the night, I would wake with muscle spasms but mentally perfectly clear and calm. Physically, I was reverberating. It felt like having a big motor in an old flivver. The running boards were shaking so hard they were in danger of falling off, along with the exhaust system, the doors and the floorboards. It was a frightening choice between operating without my accustomed processes of metaphor and shuddering to a standstill. Later I took the pills and still wrote poems and other things full of metaphors so it must have been the pain and exhaustion that were doing me in.

Every day, I went for a walk and on weekends, finally, got Chris to join me. The trails at Lemoine Point began to be familiar. At home, I would try to do my exercises and swim a bit in our little above-ground pool. The pool had been a desperation move after spending one incredibly hot summer

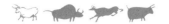

taking a course in Toronto. I should have had my head read for all the work and expense it created.

I didn't slump to the bottom until August. Under a friend's enthusiastic persuasion, I went to a concert where I was leaning forward over a balcony railing to look down at the performance on the floor. Twenty-four hours later I was suffering a lot, but when I tried getting ready for classes in September the wrecking ball hit.

The Meaning of Fibromyalgia

There should be a handbook of procedures for putting your life on hold. It should be as simple as pushing a button ...

09/90 At the start of the school year, I had been very conservative, getting Michael and Matthew to haul my boxes of stuff to school, having the caretaker arrange the room, persuading Mike and Matt to put up the bulletin board backgrounds and displays. I sat and made up daybook pages and lesson plans and class lists. I thought I was going to be okay.

I went to school one more day. By two o'clock, I had to call for someone to drive me home. My left shoulder was bent backwards so that I couldn't face forward — like a bird with a broken wing. The pain was considerable — headache, backache, neck ache, arm ache, leg ache, hand ache, foot ache ... That about covers it. Oh, I forgot the stabbing pains — everywhere there was an ache. And burning pain ditto.

I went to the physiotherapist for his advice, driving for half an hour in agony, parking the car, dragging myself into the building, waiting for the elevator, waiting in the waiting room, too pained to read a magazine — even an old magazine (talk about choices), dragging myself out, driving home again, lying down on ice packs. He advised me that I would

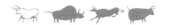

probably not be able to go to school, but this was almost an aside to the incredible effort of going to hear those few words. The appointment with my doctor was just a replay.

Then I had to make the arrangements by calling the principal and then the supply teacher. Then there was the trip to school to collect my personal belongings and show the supply teacher my carefully laid plans and materials. Every situation created its own adrenaline overload, just from the effort to overcome the pain.

By the time school started, I could barely sit up. I couldn't watch TV because I couldn't lie on either side without terrible pain in either leg. I couldn't read because it hurt my back to hold a book. I lay in bed and listened to the radio. And I worried.

To try to make sense of what was happening, I began to keep a chart which tracked headaches (how long they lasted each day — there was no such thing as a day without a headache), the treatments I was receiving, the medication I was taking, and so on. I thought that the chart would help me figure out if anything was helping or making matters worse. The chart freed me of trying to remember my progress whenever a medical person would ask me how I was. It freed me up for the worrying.

What's to worry about? Well, the specialist thought I should aim to go back the second week of October. I worried about what I could possibly do that would take the least energy and the least preparation. It was ludicrous to think of programming when even reaching for a book, writing on the board, or bending over a desk were unimaginable with the body I now had. I collected the children's comic pages from the Sunday funnies and made activities for my class out of them. It helped keep the anxiety about what I could do with the children if I was forced to go back to work. That's how much I knew about my rights as a worker.

The second week of October passed, as did the rest of

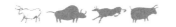

the month, in pain. The specialist's cry was, "Aim for after Christmas." I went through the same terror-provoking exercise of imagining what on earth I could do in a classroom.

Then it was, "Aim for February."

Each time I would tense as the deadline approached. Each time, I was looking right at the steamroller as it made another pass. Fortunately, before Christmas, I was given something else to worry about — money! So far, the sick leave days I had accumulated over many years of not being sick were backing me up. Now it was time for other things to start taking over.

A long time ago, when the earth was green and my dad was being eaten up by rheumatoid arthritis, I signed up for an income protection plan and promptly forgot what the ten dollars a month was for. When the school board offered Long Term Disability Insurance, I signed up for that coverage, too. By the time I was a wreck, I couldn't even remember where the policies were, let alone what to do about them.

It took a few phone calls — to the Teacher's Federation and the School Board — to get things rolling. And it took awhile to get the forms from the two companies to fill out. It took doctor's appointments to have the forms filled out. We went over what I couldn't do. We weighed my purse (two pounds) to find out the maximum I could lift.

About this time I read an article in the paper about a condition called "fibromyalgia." People who have it hurt all over. That sounded like me. I asked my family doctor if that was what I had, and she agreed that it was a strong possibility. At my next appointment with the specialist, I asked him if that was what I had. "Of course," he said. I was lucky. Criteria for fibromyalgia had just been clarified in 1990 in the American College of Rheumatology publication by Wolfe, Smythe and Yunnus. Their definition of fibromyalgia includes widespread (all four quadrants) pain existing for at least three months; and tenderness at eleven or more of the eighteen specific

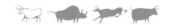

tender points on the body. Other characteristic symptoms include sleep disturbance, fatigue, morning stiffness, while common symptoms include parathsthesias, headache, anxiety reactive hypermia (trapezius muscle), and dymenorrhea. Approximately ten to twenty percent of the general population suffers from some degree of fibromyalgia, and women are ten times more likely to suffer from the disease than men. Fibromyalgia was soon after recognized as a syndrome internationally in 1992 by the World Health Organization. Before this, people had to cope with having a condition which was painfully real but not officially sanctioned, something like believing your house is haunted. It could lead to lots of disbelief.

It is one thing to know that you cannot function — and another thing to have to write down what you cannot do and then sign your name on an insurance form. It is even worse to read the descriptions by doctors of your condition. Each word in black feels like a black mark against you, no matter if your work and personal history are as white as the proverbial lily. It is depressing to see yourself labeled as "completely disabled." It may be true, but it hurts.

Christmas 1990 came, and a sorry holiday sight I was, watching everyone else decorate the tree and shop and wrap presents and cook. I just wanted to hide in a box with **DO NOT OPEN EVEN AFTER CHRISTMAS** marked on it.

Acupuncture

I did get a present that year, a wonderful one — some relief for the pain. The physiotherapist took a course in acupuncture because of several patients like myself who had intractable severe pain. For the past two years, the physiotherapist had tried a lot of things with me and on me — heat, ice, exercise of all kinds, neurostimulator, TENS®, Codatron®, manipulation, deep heat. Still I would come in, hardly able to see for the headache pain, and leave not a lot better. Pills did little but upset the rest of my system.

01/91   Like anyone else, I was partly skeptical and partly afraid and partly hopeful. I had disliked childhood vaccination needles, still dislike dental anesthetics administered with those enormous needles, and grimace when I have to have blood taken by the pleasant vampires in white. However, when a headache hit, as it did so often, anything that might help seemed like a good idea. It's hard to explain the frightening feeling that pain with no discernible end can provoke, especially when it fills your head with a gray static so that you can't even think. I sympathize with migraine sufferers.

To have the acupuncture, I had to lie down on my front on the examining table. My right shoulder and chest began

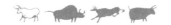

to spasm almost immediately, but I tried to ignore that in favor of hope. The first needle went in behind my left ear with a sound like the tap of a fingernail. If my headache pain was like heavy frost on a windshield, it melted in a strip on one side. When the needle went in on the right, another strip melted. A needle on the crown connected the two lateral strips. I felt as if I could see properly again!

After a few minutes of lying there letting the needles work, my right arm and shoulder were knotted painfully, shaking, but my headache was relieved. The neurostimulator applied to the painful spots completed the treatment. For the first time in two years, something was helping me.

As the weeks went on, we learned to put pillows and a heat pack under my chest to relieve the pain in the arm and shoulder. The physiotherapist used needles in various places with varying results. Sometimes a needle would sting as if it had been dipped in salt.

"Harpooning again today?" I jested. "I didn't realize I looked like a whale."

"You will keep spouting off," he replied in kind.

I guess I asked for it. Occasionally a needle would provoke a violent reaction, the muscle underneath bunching into immediate spasm. When this happened, removing the needle immediately and trying again a distance out from the spot seemed to be the best approach. Immediate removal also stopped my "Oh — ahh — oh — ah! Take it out! Take it out!"

A few situations could cause problems too — a cold draft, any urgent necessity to move (like a sneeze or a cramp), or just too long with the needles in. I suggested that a cover like the plastic dome on a deli platter would be helpful. I felt like a cube of cheese on a toothpick, so they might as well preserve me like one.

Most of the time the needles felt like just taps on the skin. The physiotherapist said that the areas around them would redden and then fade by the time he came back to

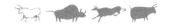

take them out. Once in a while, a spot would bleed a little when a tiny capillary was hit. The needles were disposable and the physiotherapist used rubber gloves.

There were mornings when I would be waiting at the door for the receptionist and the physiotherapist to arrive at 7:45 a.m. They could tell at a glance that I was in bad shape. The needles were the last resort when ice, heat, TENS®, and painkillers had failed to ease the terrible pain in my head.

An interesting experiment was the use of needles in headache points on my hands — in the V between index finger and thumb and on the arms, on top of the elbow. I nearly passed out that day. I began to use the TENS® on those points, twenty minutes in the morning and twenty minutes at bedtime, which seemed to give some relief as well.

It took a while to realize that the acupuncture does take away the pain but does not cure the underlying problem. What it did do was to get the pain under control so that I could do work on that problem with exercises. I have since read that experiments have shown that acupuncture causes the body to produce more of its natural painkillers or endorphins. This is different than supplying a synthetic mimic in the form of drugs.

Later on, the headaches became more confined to fleeting episodes — whenever I bent my head for more than a few seconds — and severe attacks several times a month. I also used the TENS® on acupuncture sites for insomnia — above my ankles and on my wrists — to improve my sleep.

All this time, my days were spent looking after myself. TENS® went on for twenty minutes before rising and ice packs as well, if needed. Hot showers or baths helped to release the stiffness. Stretching exercises to improve my mobility included rising on my toes, shrugging my shoulders, arm circling, torso twists, and side bends. I had to get in a rest mid-morning, noon hour, and afternoon, as physiotherapy or the doctor's appointments would allow. On good days, I tried to sit at the

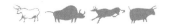

computer for a few minutes — usually fifteen minutes would be enough to wipe me out. On bad days, I lay on the couch in our living room and read murder mysteries as long as I could hold the book up. When that became too painful, I would lie in bed and listen to the radio. Bedtime meant hot bath, ice packs, and TENS®. By 7:30 p.m., I was finished.

Psychotherapy

In January, the first of my insurance programs came through. All I had to do was to have a form filled out by the doctor every two months. The waiting period for the other insurance finished in February and I was still *hors de combat* in a serious way. Now there was no question about a few months — we were looking at the rest of the year, at least.

02/91 About this time, the family doctor suggested that I go to a hypnotherapist for help in coping with the pain. I didn't like the idea. Therapists study psychology, and psychology in my university days had a lot to do with rats. Another old-fashioned and therefore deep-rooted bias against therapists is that they are for crazy people. I didn't feel that suffering tremendous pain qualified me as a rat or a crazy person. Reluctantly, I agreed to go. In order that it would be immediately apparent I wasn't and would never be a rat, I prepared a bit for the therapist. That's a "bit" not a "bite."

Appropriately, it was the first day of the war with Iraq when I went to see him. The waiting room was unusual because, instead of the omnipresent pink-and-gray silk-flower decor of specialists everywhere, the walls were wood-paneled and dark, the furniture was very worn brocade living-room stuff, classical music was playing quietly, and copies of the

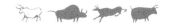

doctor's book were scattered around. Ah-ha! Another writer!

I glanced through the book, which gave examples of people with whom the doctor had worked, mainly on the premise that physical pain was exacerbated by psychological pain, and the former would be relieved by treating the latter. I was willing to try but fearful — of the doctor.

We greeted one another.

"Did you see my book in the waiting room?" he said. "It describes the kind of work that I do."

"Here is my card," I said. "It describes the work that I do and the titles of my books."

"Do you think that what I do can help you?"

"I don't know. I suppose it's possible."

"Well, you'll have to tell me a bit about yourself."

After all the people I had seen, the litany was pretty pat — mother died by her own hand after a long illness when I was eight, stepmother arrived when I was ten, father crippled with rheumatoid arthritis when I was thirteen. I started teaching at nineteen, married at twenty, extra-mural studies for degree, babies before thirty, husband bankrupt, husband seriously ill, studies for Master's degree, hysterectomy, Morton's neuroma, and ending with head lice and my bad back. My life was a therapist's delight — lots of disasters.

"You got your Master's degree to show off," he said.

You would think that would have sent me marching out of there in a feminist rage. It probably should have. My work for the degree had been motivated by a variety of things. One was a financial desire to increase my salary to hedge against my husband's possibly disabling illness and my sons' university expenses. Another was an intellectual desire to explore the thinking skills in the arts which I believed were not frills, as they are so often attacked, but vital parts of education. Showing off came a distant third, if it placed at all,

Instead of challenging him on that, my mind was on another problem. His office chair was too high to allow my

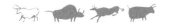

feet to touch the floor, so I was painfully braced against the legs. The pain was getting to be too much. And I said so.

"I have another chair here which seems to be very comfortable for people with bad backs," he said.

I looked at the chair, which was deep, square and upholstered in dark red naugahyde. I sat in it. It immediately tipped me back so I was looking at the ceiling. It was much better than the other chair, physically, but much worse psychologically.

"But I've already gone over my childhood in my first book," I said.

"You have to decide whether I can be of any help," he said. "I'll see you in a few days."

All the way home and for the next couple of days I bristled with indignation. Why couldn't a woman have intellectual curiosity, especially if it would increase her salary, providing a cushion in case of her partner's illness, and give some assurance that her kids could go to university if they wanted to?

He wanted an examination of my life. I'd give him an examination of my life, as it pertained to my back problem. I made a list of physical problems my back had over the years. This is a common reaction in people with serious illness. They try to go over their lives to figure out where they went wrong. I dredged up everything from my sister falling over me and wrenching my neck at age six to the surgery I had in 1984. And now the injuries around the head lice incident. Weren't these incidents sufficient to give me a pain in the back without any psychological explanation whatsoever?

Merck's Manual, a comprehensive listing of medical conditions with origins, symptoms, diagnoses, and treatments for health care professionals, has different etiologies or origins of fibromyalgia for men and women. "It is particularly likely to occur in healthy young women who tend to be stressed, tense, depressed, anxious and striving." However,

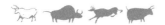

"Men are more likely to develop localized fibromyalgia in association with particular occupational or recreational strain." This bit of research may explain the peculiar dynamic between me and my therapist.

For some reason, I felt I had to be fair to the doctor and so went back once more. I sat in the tippy chair.

"Do you mind if I sit over here beside you?" he said.

"I guess not."

"Do you mind if I touch the back of your hand, like this?"

"Well, it doesn't feel very good."

"All right then, go back to when you first felt afraid."

Getting around the immediate fear of therapists and the even more immediate fear of the incapacitating pain was no easy matter, but I finally remembered something.

"I was about six and my mother had fainted while she was frying some potatoes. I tried to phone my father, which meant getting the operator on our rural line and making a long distance call to my father's business, which was two miles away. Then I tried to keep the potatoes from burning and my younger sister from getting too upset."

"You've been trying to protect yourself and others ever since," he said.

I nodded through a haze, misty-eyed, and thought, "And doing a damn fine job of it until now."

"Now try to imagine a safe place."

"At home in bed," I said. While it wasn't a painless place, at least it was a place where I didn't have to worry about therapists or anything but coping with the pain. He didn't think that was good enough?

"Isn't there any other place?" he asked. I guess he wanted a sandy beach or some more exciting locale.

"It's the place where I hurt the least," I said. And as an imaging technique it works well. I just have to imagine myself at home under the covers and I feel a bit better.

And that's where I went and stayed. If that was therapy, I

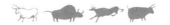

didn't want it. Much better to write a book of funny poems like *My Underwear's Inside Out*. Thank heavens for that book. Somehow I had written it before taking ill. Somehow, my friend Pat, a talented artist, had found time among her own disasters to illustrate it. Somehow I managed to do the few little revisions. Somehow it was going to be published.

I had the flutters of most authors as publication dates near. At least I didn't dream this time, as I had with my previous publication, that the books had arrived in a big box, and when we unpacked them, they were dark green with watermarked covers as though they had swum from Hong Kong instead of going by ship. It would take the whole long spring and most of the summer before any books would appear, time I used to investigate a few other ways to relieve the pain.

Meditation

Besides the meaning of fibromyalgia, one of the things I had to investigate was meditation. Most of the pain management books like *Pain: Learning to Live Without It* and so on tell you to learn relaxation techniques such as meditation and cite all kinds of wonderful case histories where meditation has helped people. A baby boomer too poor to participate in the sixties, I had always been frankly curious about meditation — and the specialist recommended it. Poets are supposed to be into stuff like meditation according to the 'image handbook' — so why not! One damn good reason why not is that working mothers have little discretionary income or time for meditation courses or anything else unrelated to earning a living and raising the family. For most of my life, the "working mother" categorization had superseded the "poet" one.

03/91 The advertisement in the newspaper first caught my attention, especially the part about the free "introductory" lecture. It was very difficult for me to go anywhere in the evening because by that time of the day my muscles were tired and making their fatigue painfully apparent. I arrived at the public library with my Obusforme® cushion in tow (at the limit of my carrying capacity) and tried to settle in a back

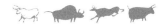

row where no one's forward view would be blocked. Perhaps the cushion seemed like an affectation to some. One lady who accompanied me to a musical evening must have thought so because she insisted we sit in mid-audience where the cushion stuck out like a sore thumb. Without the cushion, most chairs were unbearable for me after five minutes. The cushion extended my time to fifteen minutes or so if I wasn't in pain to start. Why I didn't fling myself down on the floor and scream a lot, I don't know. Maybe it would have made a difference in my treatment.

Anyway, back to the lecture on meditation. I stood up as long as possible and then submitted to the torture of sitting. The lecture went into basic principles, research results, and promotional endorsements. The only costumes to be seen were the power suits on the ladies in charge. The lecture was illustrated with overhead projections like any business seminar. Come to think of it, it was just like a business seminar with a product to sell. The time and place of the follow-up sessions were announced, and I made my painful way home, determined to give it a try.

I arrived the next Saturday afternoon in a bungalow living room, looking for oriental metaphysical signs, perhaps a fireplace tool set with multi-armed figures, or incense burning in an elephant-foot ashtray. Everything looked pretty normal, but a lot more color-coordinated than my own place which was "wait-until-the-kids-leave-home-to-redecorate" shabby. I filled out a long application form. Maybe it wasn't as much long in reality as it felt long sitting in an antique dining room chair with knobby spindles and too-high legs. All my life chairs have been the enemy. I wrote my check for two hundred dollars, a half-price bargain for the disabled. Then I waited with the mandatory posy, wilting in my lap, to be initiated. A lovey-dovey pair of newly-weds, a woman in a wheelchair, and several assorted people whom you wouldn't look at twice if they walked by on the street completed the waiting group.

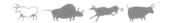

I was ushered into the den where the initiates' flowers adorned a table. A tall, thin woman of pronounced Scandinavian design examined my application, asked me impertinent questions, and told me about the mantra, a two-syllable Hindu sound, tried and true, for hundreds, nay thousands of years, for its efficacy in promoting meditation. She selected one especially for me from the many she had learned and warned me never to divulge it.

I was asked to repeat it, first aloud with the croak of someone who hasn't spoken for a bit, and then silently, with eyes closed. She gave me a little more instruction. Sit in a quiet place with a timepiece available to keep the meditation to twenty minutes. Do not make effort. Just relax and take what comes.

As usual, I made an idiot of myself by finding difficulties.

"If I can't sit because of the pain, is it all right to lie down?"

Well, no. That wasn't *maximal* position.

"What about the timing? Is it essential? I don't have a watch."

Well, yes. She thought timing was essential.

With that, I was ushered into a bedroom of the bungalow, where I could sit in an armchair undisturbed and try out the meditation. Which I did. It wasn't easy to close my eyes with the spasms in my eyelids. It wasn't easy to sit in the chair with the pains in my back and everywhere else. It was easy to do the meditation.

"How long was that?" said the sweetly-gentle lady of the house sent to retrieve me.

"About ten minutes, I'd say."

"Your time sense is quite accurate so you've probably been meditating correctly," she said.

And that was it until Monday.

At home, lying down, the meditation made me feel as if I was being rocked on long sea swells or riding a slow colorful

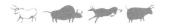

roller coaster. One of the first sessions went on for forty minutes before I could force myself to give up the restful feeling.

In a few days, back at the instructional bungalow, we were debriefed about our meditational experiences. I was told not to indulge in long sessions but to limit them to twenty minutes twice a day. There was general discussion and a video which was as close to meeting a real live Eastern guru as we would get. There were books offered. There were other courses offered. There were diets and Ayurvedic physicians offered. My worst problem was the chair I had reluctantly chosen. It was exquisitely designed for torture, and it was all I could do to keep myself from slithering off it into a nice relaxing prone position on the floor. Propriety is stiff starch to keep such misery sitting bolt (but squirming) upright.

Two more sessions, and I was licensed to meditate on my own with an invitation for a check-up any time.

Mornings now became an incredibly ponderous routine. Twenty minutes for TENS®, twenty minutes for meditation, time for a hot shower, exercises, and a walk left little time for anything else. Add a trip to the physiotherapist or doctor (for prescriptions or insurance forms) or the specialist. It is a wonder I did anything else. Mystery novels, a few minutes at the computer, feeble attempts at simple meals, the odd phone call to a friend — all helped to fill the time. With bedtime before or at eight o'clock, there weren't many lonely moments. Sometimes I would be in too much pain even to read; those times dragged until I discovered public radio (no commercials), which entertained me until the pain pills let me drift off.

It must have been a gradual process, but I began to think of my body as somehow an object apart from myself. All those times of taking off clothes to be viewed by medical strangers. All those prods and pokes which led to hours of pain. All those machines attached and discarded. All those times I had been treated as "an interesting case" or "an

Meditation

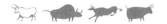

uninteresting case" or any kind of "case" must have added to the cumulative effect. It begins to seem no more personal than the family automobile being taken to the garage. A lemon of a car, perhaps.

Iridology

Early that spring, the specialist mentioned that there was a new nutritionist in town — she might be worth a try as long as I was investigating alternative therapies. "She reads your iris," he said with a shrug, half skeptical and half hopeful. So I made an appointment with the iridologist.

04/91 She was a kindly-faced blonde in a pastel gingham dress. She asked for a bit of my history. That is always the worst part of any new medical encounter. She had a box arrangement with lights and a camera and a chin rest. This was for photographing the eyes.

"Please put your chin here," she said.

I tried to bend enough. "Sorry. I can't lower my head enough." As usual, I felt ridiculous and a bit sorry for myself.

She got some thick books and propped the arrangement up until it met my chin. I looked into the box with the lights shining from the side, and she examined my irises, making notes about various brown flecks in them as she went. One meant my left leg. Another, my sweet tooth. (There's no hiding that anyway, it shows up on the hips.) To finish off, she took a picture of each eye.

"You're lucky," she said. "You have a strong constitution. Look at this picture of another person's eyes. The white lines

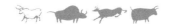

are far apart and loosely looped. Yours are tight together. This means ..."

At last, a shred of good news which I held to myself like a talisman. Then she listed the vitamins and minerals she thought I should take. But that wasn't the end. The most interesting was yet to come. Muscle testing was next.

"Raise your right arm," she said, showing me.

I tried, but winced with the pain of lifting it at all, let alone level with my shoulder.

"No problem. My daughter can help."

We went into the front of the store. I took off my watch at her direction and joined hands with her daughter, who then raised her right arm.

"First, I will test with nothing in your other hand. I'll push down to test the resistance." Which she did.

"Now, hold this bottle of vitamins in your left hand," she said, selecting from the bewildering array on her shelves. She then pushed down on her daughter's right arm.

"That seems strong for you. Now we'll determine the dosage." And she pushed down for one or two. "One is the strongest."

And so it went for Vitamin C, Vitamin E, Evening Primrose Oil, Lecithin, Calcium/Magnesium, and Zinc. Some brands were rejected as too weak or too strong or not necessary. Dosages were determined. Even my prescribed medication was tested. I was curious to see if the ones selected were the most expensive but that was not the case. I left with seven bottles worth fifty dollars, a package of green pumpkin seeds to rid me of any unwelcome microbes, and an appointment to return for the reading of the photograph.

The worst part of the recommended treatment was "the purge" — two weeks of eating gas-producing items like dried apricots, and taking a daily dose of a foul-tasting liquid that came in glass ampoules. I felt like a drug deviate, breaking them open and then hiding them in the trash. Drinking the

contents in water was one more punishment for my already well-punished self.

But the green pumpkin seeds weren't bad at all. My husband started snacking on them as proof. The vitamin and mineral supplements were just a nuisance. And the prunes which she had prescribed for constipation were a great success.

To give the whole thing the right perspective, I didn't expect supplements to cause any quick change: for years, I had been making daily salads of every raw vegetable in the refrigerator and stuffing us all with fruit for desserts. How could I be missing anything drastic? Still, illness may cause us to require more of some things for repair, I reasoned. Anyway, I took the expensive ones for a year. Since I had never learned to smoke and drank only the odd beer or glass of wine, there wasn't that to counteract.

Did the regimen make any difference? It's like measuring erosion on a rock face. If it made a difference, it's not measurable by anything I can devise. Most of the supplements were in small doses and wouldn't do any damage even if I couldn't discern any good. At any rate, it was a another distraction from the endless pain and the inability to do anything. I still have the two photographs of my eyeballs which should make for an unusual entry in the family album.

Endocrinology

I t was soon after this that the physiotherapist decided to
do something about the fact that I still couldn't bend my
head much. Most people can bend their heads so that
their chins nearly touch their chests, or at least their double
chins do. When I would try to bend my head, the closest I
could get my chin to my chest was a wide hand-span away.
This restriction made it difficult to do many simple things
like reading a book, looking a number up in the phone
book, cutting my toenails — you name it. The technique he
proposed to use involved spraying a topical anesthetic along
the muscles on either side of my spine and then gently
stretching the muscles by hand. Very slowly but surely, week
after week, I began to be able to bend my head. It was one
small victory in the midst of all the other defeats.

One week at physiotherapy, he remarked, "Your skin is
clammy again. Some days you are and some days not."

I had noticed it too and so began another chapter.
"What do you think it is?"

"Are you taking any ASA?"

"Not at the moment. It doesn't seem to do any good. Just
makes my ears ring. Could it be hormonal. I am forty-five,
after all." I thought about it and noticed that sometimes I
would wake up in a lather, too. So, back to the family doctor
for a referral to an endocrinologist. The appointment was

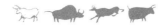

for three months hence, and meanwhile I was to fill out charts with all kinds of information. I filled them out, day by day, for the three months.

04/91 There was also the worry of being on sick leave and the worry of waiting for Long Term Disability to be approved. March 4th, the date I was eligible for disability payments, passed without a word from anyone. Then a letter arrived asking my doctor for more information. Then more waiting.

At the end of May, I called to see if there was any word, and was told that my disability application had been approved. I canceled my sick leave payments so that there would be no doubling up. Wrong move. I should have waited because nothing came at the end of June. I was getting perturbed. Finally, in the first week of July, the payment arrived and I settled up with my Board of Education for the unnecessary sick leave payments.

All wasn't sweetness and light, however, because the insurance company had made an appointment for an independent medical evaluation. It didn't seem to matter that I already had an appointment with a rheumatologist scheduled for July. Nothing would do but to have another one in August with a rheumatologist about three hours drive away. It might as well have been the moon. I couldn't drive there myself. I made arrangements for Matthew to drive me half way and Madge, my stepmother, to take me the rest.

In July, I went for my first visit with the endocrinologist. Oh joy! Internal exams are bad enough, but I had stitches in my knee which threatened to split apart if I bent my leg to put my foot in the stirrup. (I'd fallen at the post office on some uneven pavement and had to have the gash sewn up.) Breast exams are bad enough without the chest pain of fibromyalgia which makes any touch misery. All that to be told the evidence was inconclusive. I would have to have

blood tests. Then came six weeks of trotting 15 miles to the hospital once a week for blood tests. All this to find out that my hormone levels are normal. The headaches didn't seem to be following any monthly pattern.

So what about the overheating? One day while doing my exercises after a flare-up the day before, I noticed myself getting clammy after just a few repetitions. Aha! Maybe this was it! Not only was it the answer, but it also gave me another tool in judging how much to do.

As soon as I begin to overheat, I know it's time to quit, or at least rest. It has the advantage of *not* being a pain cue as well. It works whether I am exercising, trying to do some household task, or going on errands. Often with fibromyalgia, the pain does not occur immediately to warn you that you are doing something your muscles can't tolerate. The pain shows up later. Many times, having this clue about overheating has saved me from overdoing it. When I'm in a sweat, it's time to rest. I ignore the warning at my peril. Normal people work up a sweat after more prolonged exercise, but for us, a little bit can have the same effect.

About this time I began to share my discoveries and small victories with members of the local support group organized by the Ontario Fibromyalgia Association (OFA), under the umbrella of the Ontario Arthritis Association. At the support group, I was interested to find out that many of the women had gone through a variety of tests — for infection, thyroid function, and hormonal balance — for this same symptom. When I explained my theory, lights went on all over the room. If we had been Greeks sitting in overflowing bathtubs, we would have shouted, "Eureka!" What a simple thing! What a lot of misery to discover it!

Rheumatology

The first rheumatologist I met pressed me in places that hurt increasingly afterward until I was a lump of misery. Yes, I had fibromyalgia. In five years or so I might be better. Five years of this? Good grief! No one mentioned the rest of my life.

08/91 It was a blazing hot August day when I had to go for an independent medical with a second rheumatologist over three hours away by automobile. By the second leg of the trip, I was locked in an exhaustion, pain, and perspiration. When I was ushered into the examination room, I lay down on the table.

The rheumatologist came in and started asking me the routine questions. "I'm finding it hard to talk to you when you're lying down, Mrs Dawber. Would you please sit up."

"I'm finding it very hard to sit after the trip."

For the rest of the questions, I stood or rather propped myself up against the table. Physical exams for fibromyalgia patients are delightful because, in order to diagnose the condition, the doctor has to determine if certain points are painful, and, to do that, the doctor has to press on them and see if they hurt. The patient may not even be aware that these points are painful until they are pressed. The bonus is

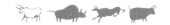

that they go on hurting long after they are pressed.

There are eighteen recognized points. Eleven have to be painful for diagnosis. I had sixteen, and by the end of the examination, they were all hurting a lot. The doctor seemed to be annoyed that she had to give the examination. It mustn't be much fun to inflict pain either.

Then there was the trip home. It is a fortunate blank in my memory and I don't even want to look it up in my journal.

It wouldn't have been so bad to have a rheumatologist confirm the diagnosis, except that I had already had the same thing done by a local specialist less than a month before. Not good enough for the insurance company! More torture!

Was the torture worth it to have my disability benefits regularized? I waited anxiously until the end of August. No payment. I waited past the first week in September. No payment. I called the company. The adjuster for my file was out of the office. The next week she was away on holiday. At the end of September, I received nothing. No money and Michael in university. I called again and the adjuster had gone home early for the day.

Phew! With no energy to get mad, I did the next best thing. The library has a book with the names of the Chairmen and Presidents of Corporations. I found the names. I wrote a letter comparing the service of the two companies with whom I was insured. My friend typed out one for the Chairman and one for the President. The letters went by courier on the Wednesday before Thanksgiving. I waited.

Friday night, when most employees would have been bound for Thanksgiving destinations, I got a call from the customer service department of the company. It was a long soothing, expensive, long-distance call that assured me that my file had been examined and my benefits approved that very afternoon and that my check would be winging its way by courier on Tuesday. Very satisfactory! I may be disabled, but I'm not powerless.

Aquabics & Tai Chi

The physiotherapist and I were now looking for something I could do in the winter for exercise. All summer I had walked every day but walking on ice or snow had caused severe flare-ups last winter. I think it is the constant adjustments your back has to make that cause the trouble. My back was just too sensitive to movement to handle the adjustments. I needed something besides my daily stretches.

10/91 What about aquabics? Removes the weight-bearing, right? I was willing to try and went back to my neighborhood pool for the first session. I explained to the instructor that I had a problem, that I might not be able to do everything, and that if I retreated to the edge to rest, to just ignore me.

After the mandatory shower, I stood on the edge of the pool, shivering, for the class to begin. The shivering was already tensing my muscles. The first few movements included raising arms, resting arms on the edge of the pool, and laying the head back in the water. That was enough to tell me that aquabics were going to mean trouble. I stayed in the water a little while, and then squeezed past the other ladies and went home, in more pain than ever and just a tad more discouraged.

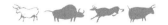

Then there was Tai Chi. The literature on fibromyalgia contains many suggestions to try Tai Chi. I dragged myself down to the community center where I found the volunteer leader with no-frills workout clothes and a kindly manner. Once again, I explained my problem and that I would just stay in the back row and do what I could.

The introductory information and demonstration were fascinating. I really wanted to be able to perform the graceful movements and build up my fitness at the same time. As always I was an eager beaver, but now an eager beaver with no teeth and a dam to repair. The first movements asked me to hold my arms up. I tried. I wanted to hold them up. I couldn't. The pain overcame. I left, a little bit more eroded, with days of pain ahead to recuperate from this feeble attempt. Not the worst part of it was that the volunteer leader was at least twenty years older.

"I've got just the thing for you!" exclaimed the physiotherapist on my next visit. "There's a physiotherapist specializing in sports injuries who has opened up a place with exercise machines. Let's try that."

So I went. I explained the problem yet again. The machines were shiny, some familiar like the exercise bicycle and the stair stepper and some unknown. The bouncy owner listened carefully and enthusiastically. She showed me how to turn the resistance of the machines down to minimum. She showed me how to use each one. Several she eliminated entirely from my routine-to-be.

The next time I went, she went around with me as I tried each one out. There were a couple of other "walking wounded" working out at the same time, all of us with major difficulties. I had on my old red track suit for comfort. I got around at the minimum and congratulated myself.

Two days later I went back and, interested in the music, the chatter of the therapist, the progress of the other exercisers, I forgot to check the resistance of a machine. Major

mistake. I went home to ice packs and waited days until I was well enough to try again. And again. And again.

By November, the physiotherapist and I were both tired of damage control and gave up on the machines.

"It seems to me that my weakest areas are always breaking down. What if I just do an exercise that would work those muscles? Forget about the stronger ones for now?"

He wrinkled his brow and thought for a moment. I felt responsible for some of the height and wrinkles of that brow.

"I've got an idea," he said. "Just a minute."

He came back with a piece of stretchy material that I hoped would change my life, for the better. The stuff looked like a wide flat strip of balloon material. It was called Theraband®.

"Get your husband to tie one end of this on the shower rod. Tie a bit of dowel on the loose end. I want you to pull down with both hands, just once. We'll see what happens."

What happened was that I could do it. We had finally found a baseline exercise which did not make things worse but worked the sore areas very gently. Eureka!

This is not to say I was better. Carrying three jars of jam did me in one day. Anything over two pounds had that effect. I would end up parked at the Physiotherapy Clinic before their eight o'clock opening, my head splitting, in need of acupuncture for some relief.

The headaches were muscle spasms right up my back, up my neck, over my skull and even to my eyelids. They had the effect of diminishing my eyesight, my mental functioning, everything, to a gray mass of pain.

Throughout the early months of 1992, I cautiously increased the exercises, one repetition a day. When I got to six, my condition flared up. I waited two weeks for the flare to pass and began again. One repetition. Then one repetition in each of four rounds of my stretching exercises. Then two repetitions in each round. Every time I built up to a certain point,

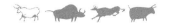

a flare would knock me backward. I would start again, one repetition at a time.

We added a pull-up exercise using the Theraband® once more with dowels on the ends. It took three months to be able to do twenty repetitions of the first exercise and three more months to be able to do twenty repetitions of the second. In the meantime, other things were happening. My husband won an award from his company and part of the prize was a three-day cruise in the Bahamas.

Like many people, our holidays had been mostly of the camping-with-the-kids variety. Once we had gone to Mexico for a week. It was a never-to-be-forgotten experience. A cruise in the Bahamas seemed too good to pass up, but could I do it? I could barely tolerate the hour's drive to my stepmother's.

I investigated travel aids and found an inflatable neck pillow and another inflatable pillow to put on my lap to support my arms. I found that my orthopedic bed pillow would fit in the bottom of our suitcase. We decided to try it.

One problem was the meal schedule. If I had the early dinner, I had to have the early breakfast, and I needed more time in bed than that allowed. If I had the late dinner, I would miss it because I would be in bed before the sitting. Since breakfast buns and coffee were available on deck, we went with early dinner and missed the regular breakfast. Dinners were too good to pass up!

I managed the trip to the airport, the airport itself, the plane trip, and the airport in Miami, but by the time I got to the ship I just wanted to lie down for a good long time and I did. The only exception was the reception where my husband was honored for his work. I wouldn't have missed that for ten bad backs.

When the ship (which looked as though a whale had taken to dive bombing and been stuck amidships) docked in Nassau, we were tempted by all the guided tours. Most of

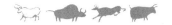

them lasted far too long for me to contemplate. What we did turned out to be much more entertaining, a hired car with a driver who was a marketing student definitely in the right career path. I got to see the schools and my husband got to see the historical points. And when my back started to wear out, we went back to the ship for another rest.

Back in Florida, we did the same thing to see the Everglades. Every morning, we were able to go for a walk in a small state park with, wonder of wonders, paved pathways perfect for perambulating wrecks who couldn't walk on sand. The warm sun made me feel almost human after a winter of mall-walking.

The last night, we watched in amazement as the planes carrying students on spring-break flew in an endless stream out of the overcast northern sky into Miami. We were glad to be going home and glad that I had managed so well. Not in a partying mode but in a low-key sort of lazy mode. I have an image of fibromyalgics moving a bit like Queen Elizabeth, slowly, with dignity, smiling gently but minus the waving. A weighted-at-the-bottom way of moving.

The only disaster happened on the way home at the airport in Toronto. My husband was carrying a shopping bag for another company couple while they made a dash for whatever. He set the bag down and was rewarded with the tinkle of two forty-ounce bottles of duty-free vodka breaking into wet splinters. It would have taken more than that to dampen our triumph on holiday, even if it was more like one for an eighty-year-old in poor health. Back to the regimen.

Insurance Inquisition

Even though I had been approved for disability by two insurance companies, that didn't mean the end of worry. Every two months, a form had to be filled in by my doctor for one company. That necessitated an appointment and, when user fees were applied to such forms, I had to pay for having the form filled out. As if that wasn't enough, the same company surprised me one morning with a visit from two detectives. I was so amazed that I didn't even ask for identification. Luckily, Michael was home from university, so I wasn't alone.

11/92 "You're lucky, ma'am. The company said you were an upstanding citizen so we didn't have to stake you out."

All they did want was to look at my prescriptions, my exercise equipment, my records, and so on for more than an hour. I had to relate the whole tale again from the beginning ... and spell big words like "fibromyalgia" and "amitriptyline." These people were not familiar with the condition and had no medical background. They were, as they said, private investigators.

How would they know anything more than what had already been reported by two G.P.s, a physiotherapist, and five specialists? Seemed like a waste of time and money to me.

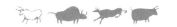

They assured me that lots of people try to get disability money fraudulently. Those people must be masters of deceit. They assured me that some doctors help people submit fraudulent claims. Then why is it so hard to find serious treatment if you are sick? Beats me.

All distractions aside, I was working on my exercises every day and going for my walks and having acupuncture once a week for pain control. My routine took up a large part of my day.

It wasn't until I tried a combination muscle relaxant and painkiller (Robaxacet®) that I got any relief. It didn't help if a headache was already underway. If I took one before a necessary but headache-causing activity (like riding in the car to visit or going out to dinner), I could sometimes last longer. Eventually, however, spasms made lying down the only relief.

And lying down isn't much of a relief if you have to sleep with pillows tucked under your legs and ice packs gradually losing their cool down your back.

When Christmas 1992 rolled around, there was a big difference, I felt. I didn't bake a single cookie. I knew better than to waste valuable energy on something that could just as easily be bought. I didn't decorate the house, but when it came time for the men to put up the Christmas tree, I watched with unaccustomed pleasure because I wasn't hurting quite so badly. Christmas dinner wasn't quite the nightmare of the previous four. It didn't take me all week to recuperate. Mind you, I was tired, not flattened, by the time Michael and Matthew headed back to university.

But what had I achieved since first being stricken with back pain that day in 1988, over four years ago, when the head lice infested my school and home? Long term disability for a condition so new that the insurance company had trouble spelling the name. Temporary relief from chronic pain by taking muscle relaxants. The knowledge that a host of therapies from acupuncture through psychotherapy to yoga

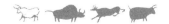

offer no lasting hope. But next to no knowledge of the cause, let alone a cure, for my illness. The medical and health community seemed as puzzled by my illness as I was. I feared I would have to resign myself to this fate, giving thanks for those few days, like Christmas 1992, when I could breathe without acute pain, but not live anything like a full life as a mother, wife, and teacher. There had to be something more I could do.

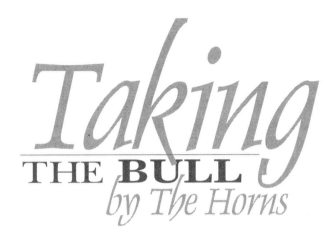

Taking
THE **BULL**
by The Horns

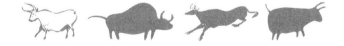

Making Metaphors

In 1993, I began to have a life again. True, it was still dominated by exercises, walks, TENS® treatments, acupuncture, and doctor's appointments, but there were moments. Some mornings, I woke up without pain and it lasted until I moved a muscle. Some days, I could stay up until ten o'clock or go out for dinner with friends and actually enjoy it. Other days when I started a new exercise or had a mishap, it was game over.

One very unusual thing happened. My vision changed. Ever since I had hurt my back, my left eye had seen the world with an annoying yellowish shadow. I had mentioned this to my doctor and she didn't have any suggestions except to have my eyes checked, which I did. Nothing wrong. The physiotherapist had run into the problem a few times with whiplash patients.

One morning, I was washing my hair under the tub faucet and noticed that when I bent over, it relieved the pain in my chest a bit. Doing my exercises, I would stop when the pain mounted and curl up in a ball. The pain would lessen a bit. At physiotherapy that week, I was lying on my stomach looking through the hole in the bench at the carpet when I realized that I was seeing it all in the same color, with both eyes. The visual anomaly had disappeared and has not come back. Weird!

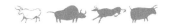

Michael graduated from university in June, and with careful planning of pills, rests and opportunities to stretch, I made it two hours by car, three hours at the ceremony, a short time at the reception, dinner at a restaurant, and the two hours home. The only part that was truly miserable was the trip home which no amount of pills could ease.

08/93 August of 1993 was unusual in several ways. The weather was beautiful after a couple of years of unpleasant Augusts. I was in good shape and making good progress with my exercises. I was optimistically looking forward to going back to work in September of 1994. Surely one more year should set me right.

Then I fell apart. One evening getting supper, Michael had made a little applesauce in our old pressure cooker. While he was busy dishing up the rest of the food, I automatically snapped open the cooker to put the two cups of sauce into a dish. After I opened it, I stopped in horror. It had been years since I had even thought of doing such a 'strenuous' thing. It was a measure of how normal I was feeling that the old appraising interior alarm had not stopped me.

Nothing hurt, so I cautiously went and sat down while the men finished the serving up. That evening, the tiny reading group to which I belonged was scheduled to meet for the first time that fall. I went. And sat on a card table chair. And shared a book with someone else, leaning over to read.

The next morning I was a little stiff but nothing dramatic, so I just did all my precautionary routines and went to visit a friend's class as had been arranged. I read some poems, holding the book up. I looked down at the student's writing. And then I went to my regularly-scheduled physiotherapy appointment.

It didn't seem like an out-of-the ordinary flare-up until Friday when I got a headache at the garage where I was

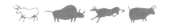

waiting for servicing of my car. Still, that wasn't a big deal. I could ice that and take a pill.

Saturday, even though I was stiff, we went to a restaurant for dinner with friends. During the dinner, my head gradually drifted down to meet my right shoulder. Everyone kept talking, but I shut up and listened, trying to figure out what was happening in my back. By the time we got home, I knew it was World War Back revisited.

I tried pills, ice, TENS®, meditation, pillows (under, on, beside and almost-ready-to-eat). My husband decamped to the empty bedroom. I rocked myself until overload mercifully knocked me out.

The next day, I was hurting, but I had hurt before, so we went for a walk. By the time we got home it was as if a finger on my right hand had been stuck in a light socket. A string of pain lights was flashing all the way from my neck to my fingertips. Chris went to the drugstore for replacement cold packs, and I rotated five of them until they were warm and went on to ice in zip lock bags.

On Monday morning, Chris drove me in to physiotherapy for the 8 a.m. opening. Acupuncture, neurostimulator, ice — I was still gritting my teeth and trying not to whimper when I left.

And that's the way it stayed for two weeks. I couldn't cut my food. I couldn't hold a pen. I couldn't turn over in bed. I woke up in the same position, on my back, as when I went to sleep. It hurt to lie down, so I spent every day sitting in a nest of pillows, rotating ice packs and trying to read every mind-numbingly-light book I could get. My right arm was knotted with the spasms. Perhaps this is what it is like to be struck by lightning — a lightning bolt lasting three weeks!

All this time, I worried about the result of this attack. Would I have lost all the strength I had built up so painfully over two years? I tried to do a few stretches but realized that I couldn't tell the effect because the pain was already too

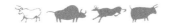

bad. Not a good move. Even a five minute walk was torture.

In three weeks, I began to do better. The pain retreated from the forearm to the elbow with just forays out to remind me. I began to hold my head up a bit straighter. I began to do a few stretches successfully. I began to get bitchy. I was so tired. Pain is tiring.

It was six weeks, all told, before I was back to square one. Square one was not, as I feared, two years back, but back to where I was in September. Not quite back to September because now I knew the third place in my back which could cause problems and, roughly, how it was triggered. The physio-therapist and I also knew where to go with the exercises. The *latissimus dorsi* needed work to stabilize the raising of my arms.

So, to work with the Theraband®. The new exercise was a one-armed pull down. I dutifully did one on each side one morning when I was feeling chipper. By mid-afternoon the headache had hit and I was taking Robaxacet® and applying ice. When that didn't work, I tried the TENS®. The head-ache subsided a little — until the middle of the night when I had to go through the whole thing again. A bad back is a lot like a baby in its effects on sleep, independence, and life in general.

The next day was physiotherapy anyway, so I hung in until then. The pain centered in the T8 area (eighth tho-racic vertebra) and felt like a hot fist despite all my atten-tions. After the acupuncture, I felt unaccountably weepy and it may have just been the relief from the pain. I do every-thing backwards — giggle at funerals and cry at celebrations.

Through all this I kept in mind that story of the farmer who gave his son a calf: "Son," he said, "lift this calf every day and, as it slowly grows bigger, your muscles will become stronger and stronger. By the time you and the calf grow up, you will be able to lift a whole bull." Damn it — I wanted to take the bull by the horns and resolve this dilemma. Well, I'm not sure whether the lifting part or the bull part of this

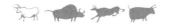

story is more appropriate to being a fibromyalgic. Where the horns fit, wear them.

Suddenly I was able to make metaphors again, to look at my condition from an objective point of view, not obscured by my pain. I was at last able to move through the impasse of my medical dilemma, where I was offered a series of choices for treatment which proved unacceptable, if not downright injurious to my health. I could now take this bull by the horns, to use the age-old figure of speech and logic or argument. Liberating metaphors began to flow, offering me the courage to seek alternative forms of treatment for my medical problems.

A runner crouches in the blocks before the sprint, concentrating on readiness, waiting for the starter's gun to send the muscles into smooth powerful action. From the time of my injury, I have had a recurring image/daydream of myself as that runner.

Five years ago, in my dream, I always collapsed at the starter's gun, as if felled by the sound. I was always unable to rise, feel strength or sense the readiness for muscle action. At times even a crouch was totally unimaginable. As time went on, I began to be able, in my mind at least, to hold the crouch with a sort of ghost of myself rising and taking the first steps in the race. The feeling of the muscles, smoothly flexing to do this, comes as a bodily memory of the way I used to be. It also represents a profound desire to feel that way again.

Benchmarks

I am doing wonderfully well. I had a whole good month in July. I decide to begin a new exercise — pulling toward myself with the Theraband®, tied to the doorknob, with one hand. I have already been pulling 32 repetitions with hands together. I manage to increase to three with each hand. Then disaster hits. In the night I feel the old stabbed-in-the-back pain. Physio calms it down, and I put off exercises for a couple of days.

Cautiously, I ease back into exercises leaving the pullback strictly alone for a week. Everything's feeling okay, so I decide to try half the Theraband® width for one repetition. Again it spasms in the night.

I wait another two weeks, into September. Surely this will be enough rest. I try one repetition one day and wait a day. It doesn't seem too bad, so I try again the third day. No go, so I give up on it and decide to go with what I can do. Maybe this is the limit for me. I am disappointed. Especially since my rehabilitation plan has to be reviewed by the specialist and me. We have to decide to scrap it. I just won't possibly be ready by January. Disappointment.

Near the beginning of October, my neck locks. I don't panic but jump in a hot shower, take a Robaxacet, and lie down with an ice pack. It doesn't get worse and gradually fades after a few days.

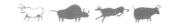

Thanksgiving and Matthew is home bringing two apartment mates who are too far from home for weekend visits.
It's beautiful outside and I go out on the deck and look at
the last roses before supper. A stray weed bothers me so I
casually give it a tug. Wrong move.

I'm up and down in the night with ice packs and
Robaxacet®. It's a good thing Chris is a capable cook because
he ends up cooking the turkey. I try to help and put on a
cheerful face for guests though I feel as if I'm the turkey.

When they all leave the next day, I'm feeling better and
decide to do one round of exercises to loosen up. Unfortunately, a Theraband® snaps and gives me a jolt. I'm on ice
again. From there it is all downhill. My specialist and I decide
to consult the pain specialist again. I ask to be put on the cancellation list.

11/94 November 10, 1994 — I will remember this day for
a long time. The pain specialist's office calls with an appointment available after lunch. I quickly arrange for Chris to
take me. I'm not sure what shape I'll be in afterward — able
to drive or not.

The pain specialist remembers me from three years ago.
We talk while dread for the examination builds. Then I'm
being poked and prodded. I want to be able to say where the
pain is, exactly, as he requires in order to do anything, but I
can't say. However, I almost faint. Twice.

The specialist figures that it is apprehension, but I'm not
so sure. It is the same overheating effect I get when I lift my
arms or do one repetition too much. He waves aside my
explanation and chuckles pleasantly. Pleasant for him. He
asks me if I want him to try the injection. I ask him what he
would advise his wife. He says he would tell her to go home
and try two things — Toradol® at the first twinge, a hot
shower and, if there is still a problem, another Toradol®. He

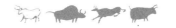

cautions me about the stomach-eating side-effects of the medication.

We leave. I expect to be sore. I'm not. I'm feeling strangely euphoric. My shoulder blade area feels peculiar. It has felt that way since the specialist prodded it. After supper, I take the unusual step of calling a friend and going out to the mall for something on a special sale. We both buy sweaters. I go to bed pleased with myself but puzzled.

In the morning, I move as I wake and feel pain in the mid back. I experiment with positions, trying to duplicate the pressure of the previous day's prodding. I find a position that gives relief, but I don't have long to stay there because I have an appointment with the physiotherapist to discuss yesterday's results. On the drive in, each time I feel a twinge in the mid back, I am able to relieve it with a twitch of my shoulder. I explain what has happened and the physiotherapist is disappointed that the pain specialist could do nothing but happy that I am able to find relief. He examines the back.

"This is remarkable!" he says. "The tightness down the left side is gone. The muscles feel flexible for the first time in six years."

"I feel like leaping up and cheering!" And I do too.

"Think it but don't do it," he smiles.

He is able to identify the sore spot and treats it for the first time with diathermy. We agree that I restrict myself to stretches and leg Theraband® exercises. For the rest of the week, I try to do this, increasing one round a day until I get to three rounds and stay there for a couple of days but I run into problems.

The shoulder is not calmed easily any more. I cut back to just stretches. The physiotherapist and I agree to consult the regular specialist. There is a cancellation next day.

I explain what has happened. He examines it. He has me twist my hand.

"The serratus posterior inferior," he says. "It's a tough

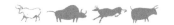

one." The exercise he gives is to grip the edge of the table, just once for a couple of seconds. And he recommends a figure eight bandage to take the pressure off.

Next day at physiotherapy, I am trussed up with the stretchy bandage around the front of each arm and crossing on my back. It cuts into my armpits but gives me immediate relief from a headache which was developing. Wow!

For the next week I wear the bandage eight hours a day and have friction abrasions in my armpits. I'm going to be the only woman in the country with callused armpits! But it seems to help.

The relief is so transitory, however, as to be a figment of my imagination. Soon I can barely close my hand without the serratus going into a spasm. I can't work at the computer. I can't do much in the kitchen. I can't do any exercises. I can only walk five minutes before the serratus goes into spasm. I can't even sit up and read even with the book on pillows. I am terrified. Here I am back four years, lying listening to the radio. I can't even hold the phone to talk to a friend. The Toradol® doesn't provide much relief even though my family doctor raises his eyebrows and says that it is as powerful as a shot of morphine.

What terrifies me most is that I don't know if it will take years to rebuild or what. My husband quietly advises me to apply for my Teachers' Disability Pension which entails application forms for the doctor to fill out once more. I go and do it. At that moment the possibility of ever being well enough to teach is remote indeed.

Soon the old determination kicks in. I will listen to tapes or watch videos or create into a tape recorder, but I will not give up no matter how long it takes. The physiotherapist and I discuss the situation and decide I have no choice but to do only what the serratus will allow and that just means daily living activities, no exercises for awhile.

A week before Christmas, Michael moves into the first

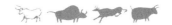

place of his own. I want so much to go with the guys. I prepare myself carefully, bandage, Robaxacet®. While the three of them are loading the truck, I assemble lunch so I won't be tempted to touch a thing. For the first time in six weeks, I make a very simple salad. I can just barely cut the onion if I do not grip it but hold it down with my arm.

I survive the hour's ride by wedging my left hand under myself to counter any forward pull. The roads are rather bad but we make it. The men hook up the stove first so the lasagna (store-bought) can keep warm. While the men unload the truck, I wash enough plates and flatware for the meal. Michael is over the moon with having his own space, even if it is an old mobile home back in the bush. A writer's haven — cheap and fully-equipped with major appliances. We eat and prepare to leave him to it. Chris has to drive the rental truck which is standard transmission and Matt will drive me in the car. That is we will if Chris can find the keys. I walk around outside with my eyes on the slush, looking for a glint of metal. The rest search the boxes and drawers and bags and so on.

After half an hour we give up and decide we'll have to pick up the truck tomorrow with the spare set of keys. Chris is not amused. Matt drives us home. I am scrunched into the back seat beside the coolers which held lunch. An hour later we pick up the keys with embarrassment. Chris is not amused at having to pay for an extra day either. At home, I am feeling fairly perky so I make a quick wipe of the coolers before Matt takes them downstairs. And there are the keys!

By Christmas, I can hang decorations and tinsel on the tree. The first time in five years. I wrap presents and can do it. I peel potatoes for Christmas dinner using sponges held on with elastics as supports for my arms. Michael, Matt, Chris, Madge, Barbara and a cousin come for dinner and I enjoy it.

By New Year's 1995 I can walk for 15 to 20 minutes. I decide to try one repetition of each stretch and one grip of

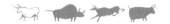

the table with each hand. I can do it. The next day I begin again but as I stretch out the Achilles tendon, it pains sharply.

By the time I get back to physiotherapy the next week, the heel and calf are really sore and I have to give up walking, stairs, and exercises. I could scream, but I gather mystery novels and sit, with ice on the heel and leg, and read until I could care less whodunnit ever again. Three weeks to three months it could take.

In minimum time, it is improving rapidly. I start again. Very cautiously. In February, I have ten days when I cannot exercise, whereas in January it was nineteen days.

Every week I have a new "first." One day in January, I can get supper by myself. A few weeks later, I can do the dishes as well. A couple of weeks after that I get groceries by myself but leave them in the car for Chris to carry in. A couple of weeks later I can carry them in a bit at a time. The week after Christmas, I can make my bed. The next week, I can change my bed. The week after that I can change both beds. The week after that Matthew comes home and so I do three beds.

One week, I can carry a small load of wash, bundled in my arms and held close, downstairs to the washer and put it in. Chris has to get it out for drying and folding. The next week, I can get it out of the dryer and fold it. The next week, I can get it out of the washer. Soon I can do two or three loads. I still can't manage the laundry basket though.

I go to school to read poems, but bending to look at the students' writing stirs up my back and the next day, the headache hits. I remember the bandage and swear to the physiotherapist that I will wear it the next time. I do and there is no headache next day, but I'm tired out. The next time, I'm not so tired.

When we get a wonderful mild week for March break, one of my teacher friends calls to ask me to go for a walk. I go with her to the park. I have been walking on the road where there is clear and firm footing. This will be the first time into the

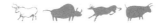

park and I'm a little afraid. The sun is glorious. The trails are wet, muddy and in some places slushy or icy. I pray a lot and watch my feet. We are almost around when we are confronted by a long snowy stretch. I can't see any way around it, but my muscles are tiring. I'm almost through when the snow gives and my foot turns a bit too far. The Achilles lets me know it. I head for home and ice packs and the whole nine yards.

My lower back ache, my legs ache, my foot pains, but I now have a benchmark, a reality check. I'm not up to par yet but I'm heading in the right direction. And this time, I don't feel hobbled. Before that day back in November, my back had always felt as if something was too short in there. Now it isn't. The difference in my head is remarkable too.

For a month I have not had a headache and the weird electrical activity has decreased a lot: the shocks that would lift me off the bed when I was lying down, accompanied by flashes of light inside my eye and booms in my ears, replaced by a writhing feeling at the bottom of my spine, then at the top of the spine a feeling as if my head was wreathed in a sting of pulsing lights; then later the whole spine would feel as if it were writhing, like a snake with a rake holding it down in the middle. Light effects accompanied this but no sound. The writhing gradually diminished, and with it, the lights. Now there are only flickers when I have relapses, with pulsing along the spine.

When I read about the discovery of new tissue connecting the muscles of the neck and shoulders to the dura, the covering of the brain and spine, I thought this might lead to an understanding of my condition. I watched in health magazines and medical journals for any tidbit of information that could have any bearing, however remote, on my situation.

Nutritional Therapy

When I was a child, I took cod liver oil. I can still remembering burping the ghastly stuff through my morning classes in high school. If I had only known! Prenatally, I took iron. Apart from that I hadn't really looked into vitamins until I fell ill.

05/95 In that first year off work, I went to the nutritionist and took her regimen of a superduper multivitamin and other things but I gave up after about a year. If I had only known! I will be thinking that a lot in the next pages so I'll try to refrain from repeating it out loud.

An acquaintance, originally from Toronto, told me about the doctor she was seeing there. She was having some luck treating her chronic fatigue problems. Out of desperation, or more romantically, prescience, I called up and made an appointment. I was instructed to write down my complete medical history and to arrive fasting. The latter was definitely easier to do than the former. Childhood diseases, operations, childbirth, the whole history of the back problem — the lot occupied several days of effort. What was important in all this?

When the day came and I had to take the train for the more-than-two-hour trip to the city, I wasn't sure I was up to the challenge. I had to navigate my way through unfamiliar

territory, take the subway, and then walk, carrying my load limit of Obusforme® cushion and folding footstool, both of which were necessary for me to bear the train. It was a bit foolhardy in my condition. However, fools rush in. Unknown to me, the fasting probably helped me get there as much as anything.

More paperwork greeted me upon arrival. Paperwork of the kind I hate most — boxes to check off whether I was 'greatly', 'somewhat' or 'not at all' whatever. There was a questionnaire on diet. There was a questionnaire on lifestyle. That one could have been answered in one phrase, 'Don't have one any more — life or style.' I wasn't impressed, but it kept me busy while I waited, and distracted me a little from the pain.

The interview with Dr. M, however, was a different story. She actually looked over my history carefully and asked questions. Certainly this was the first time a doctor had interacted with me in that way. Many times, I had been either not asked or cut short, but seldom conversed with as if I had some worthwhile information. Of course, many of the previous doctors were specialists who were looking for a pattern that corresponded to their own specialty. Dr. M was not a specialist in that way. In fact she was a General Practitioner. "Four Star" General Practitioner!

The interview took quite some time. I was introduced to Dr. M's friendly assistant, who took the required blood and urine samples, and I was advised to go get something to eat and have a rest, which I did. And that was it for the first visit — except for paying four hundred dollars for the tests not covered by provincial insurance.

Lighter in body and pocketbook but somehow in mind too, I made my way home to wait the month before the next visit.

The second trip was no less painful but less nerve-wracking because I was at least familiar with the route and the people at my destination. On arrival, I was given the results of my tests

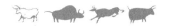

and questionnaires. It was lot a lot to read, but hey, this was a waiting room, and it sure beat the usual reading material. Maybe a clear answer would emerge from the printouts. They certainly taxed my brain. The analyses of blood, urine, diet, and lifestyle seemed to give lots of contradictory conclusions. I was disappointed. How could anything be made of all this?

Ahh! That's where the art of medicine comes in — and the skill and experience of the practitioner. Not all are created equal. Dr. M went over everything with me, quickly noting what seemed significant to her. She recommended a list of vitamins and minerals — vitamin A and D in cod liver oil (my old friend), vitamin B complex, vitamin C to bowel tolerance (take as much as will give diarrhea and cut back onc), vitamin E and evening primrose oil for essential fatty acids, magnesium, and a multimineral. That about covered all bases. Oops no! A digestive aid to help absorb all this, and acidophillus to help populate the bowel with friendly bacteria. And a course of anti-yeast medication. Oh, and Dr. William Crook's anti-yeast diet, which means no sugar, no yeast, no additives. And a vitamin B-12 shot and a magnesium sulfate intravenous on the way out. Phew!

The magnesium injection was a new experience. Dr. M's assistant warned me that I would taste it in my mouth and possibly feel as if I was going to wet my pants, but that this injection might help a lot. I tasted it. I didn't wet my pants. I didn't feel any particular effect. I paid for my shots, walked across the road to the pharmacy, and went home. The next day, I buzzed around like a mad-assed fiend. And then the effect wore off. I wore out and that was that.

Suddenly, I was taking thirty capsules, pills, tablets, etc. a day. I had to make a schedule just for the supplements, which wasn't as easy as it sounds. Don't take minerals with bran, so not at breakfast. Take acidophillus on an empty stomach. Digestive aid at meals. Take vitamins and minerals at different times as they compete in the absorption process.

Nutritional Therapy

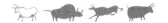

Don't take the multimineral at bedtime as it might be too stimulating then. Take Evening Primrose oil three times a day. Take the anti-yeast medication four times a day. Take the multimineral and magnesium twice a day. Take the vitamin C as often as you can. Even the experts disagree on the optimum procedures.

Shopping for the supplements was another adventure. Remember — my new diet calls for no sugar, no yeast, no additives. Check out the labels on the supplements. Not all are created equal here either. Some have sugar. Some have yeast. Some have coloring. There are all sorts of components possible — rosehips, carob powder, alfalfa, you name it! Some ingredients, I was horrified to learn, are not even listed on the label. Coal tar is an example. In addition, minerals come in many different formulations which are not equally-well absorbed. Magnesium is a good example. Calcium another. Dr. M recommended citrate forms, i.e. magnesium citrate, calcium citrate, etc.

Some supplements I could not get in Kingston, so I experienced the interesting world of mail-order nutrients. Everything from a one-a-day multivitamin to shark cartilage and the latest exotic herb is available a phone call away. Inspirational books and alluring unguents added to the catalog.

I had enough to cope with so I stuck to the boring old vitamins and minerals. Betain de hydrochloride with pepsin, my recommended digestive aid, was as much of a frisson as I could afford.

Sixty dollars a month about did it. Two dollars a day? If you've given up coffee, a muffin, a soft drink, a chocolate bar, or a bag of chips and substitute the supplements, you'll come out even financially — and way ahead nutritionally. It's way cheaper than smoking or drinking. Not as glamorous perhaps but it certainly gives you something to do — figuring out when to take what.

At that second appointment with Dr. M in August 1995,

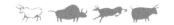

she recommended a diet as well as supplements. The diet was from Dr. Wm. Crook's book, *Chronic Fatigue and the Yeast Connection.* This despite little Candida on my test results. The reason becomes apparent as you study the diet. By banning sugar and yeast, it eliminates almost anything processed and, in this way, additives which strain the body's detoxification processes.

Doing without sugar and yeast sounded simple until I went shopping and started reading labels. I was mostly all right in the fruit and vegetable section except I put back the cantaloupe because those melons are the most susceptible to mold. I also dropped the salad dressing and croutons. Sugar and yeast in those.

Bread and cheese? Pass. Sugar and yeast in bread. Bacterial culture in cheese.

The meat section is better except for deli meats. Drop that barbecued chicken. Forget bacon and ham — too many additives. Fresh meats are okay.

On to the dairy case — butter, milk, and yogurt, allowed, as long as the yogurt is unsweetened.

Frozen foods? Plain fruit and vegetables. Avert my eyes from the ice cream, Mexican and Chinese specialties and fruit juices. Even "pure" juices seem to have sugar added in some "-ose" form or other — sucrose, dextrose, fructose, maltose, you-name-it.

What about the center of the store. Mostly, forget it. Oh, I can go for a tin of tuna or salmon, in plain water. Pasta — whole-wheat, or rice — whole grain, perhaps.

I just saved a bundle. No junk food, no soft drinks, no cookies, no ice cream. All of the stuff that costs more per pound than steak. I just saved time, except for reading labels and putting down things in disgust. Imagine! Canned soup has sugar and yeast in it as prime ingredients. Who'd-a-thunk-it?

However, when I get home, I have to rethink everything.

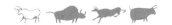

Make my own salad dressing with lemon juice (No vinegar allowed!) and olive oil and herbs. Raw garlic turns out to be a girl's best friend — giant yeast killer and, most importantly, something with flavor that's on the approved list. Pepper turns out to be toxic. The herbs are in for a workout!

For the first three days of the diet, I cough and don't feel very well. It's supposed to be the effect of the yeasts dying off from lack of sugar in the body. Their decaying remains are toxic and have to be processed on through. A friend, also newly on the diet, coughs and feels punk for two weeks. After the initial hurdle, we both start feeling a bit better. If we didn't feel like killing for a chocolate bar, we'd be better yet. If our families didn't think we were nuts, we'd be even better. If we didn't have to cook every last crumb from scratch — no more pizza — we'd be even better. Meals begin to look like those from my childhood in the fifties. However, it seems like a healthy thing, a logical thing to do. Why didn't we do it before? I guess because the focus was always on the pain and no one suggested a link between pain and nutrition.

My former diet would not have led anyone to suspect anything wrong there. For thirty-five years, I'd been making salads every night for supper, cooking vegetables and having mainly fruit for dessert. There were cookies and soda pop and chips but quantities and occasions were always limited. Pizza or something fast came in once a week, but I drew the line at fried chicken and chips. Too much grease and not enough nutrients. Expensive malnutrition.

I always liked chocolate, though. It made me feel good, in small amounts. Since I didn't react well to coffee, tea, or booze, it seemed a small vice.

You would think my husband would scream at my new diet, but no, he was having problems with high blood sugar and had been cutting way down on sugar anyway. Since I wasn't bringing any into the house, it helped him kick the sugar habit too. With walks for exercise and the diet, his

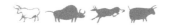

blood sugar began to stabilize at more normal levels. My sons, however, didn't take as kindly to the change, and meals and shopping began to take on a double-barreled burden — cook and shop for myself and, when they were home, cook and shop for them. Since I often could not do much of either, I often had to take it one day or one meal at a time. Again Chris willingly filled in the gaps, did the major shopping and when I couldn't, cooked whatever I prescribed.

The "goop" diet was my husband's term for the metabolic clearing diet. The "goop" was a hypo-allergenic mix of nutrients which were supposed to aid your body in the detoxification process. It was not cheap. Sixty-five to a hundred dollars a can, depending on the brand. A can would last about 10 days. Dr. M offered a consolation: "You'll save on groceries."

The "goop" was a powder to be mixed with water or juice in a blender to make a "shake." Since I couldn't have fruit juice, the only way I could bear to drink it was to add a banana or a few strawberries to the blender and then use a straw to avoid tasting as much as possible. Chris sampled it, liked it, and joined me on this diet.

I gagged down the first three days worth and then began to add in foods — mostly rice and vegetables — as per the instructions.

For the first few days, I felt extremely well — the best I had felt in a long time. Well enough to begin decreasing my medication, the abhorred amitriptyline. I managed to shave 5 milligrams off the dose without causing major upset. At the end of two weeks, I felt great ... weak but great. Chris felt well too.

Reading To Heal

I began to feel so well that I tried to drive for a couple of hours to my next appointment with Dr. M. But by the time I got home, my back was hurting again — and it kept on hurting, until …

09/95 Dr. M suggested another book to read, *Wellness Against All Odds* by Dr. Sherry Rogers, which had to be ordered directly from the publisher. My copy arrived and I became immersed in the world of nutritional therapies — varieties of diet, allergies causing everything from rashes to — Eureka! — back pain. Dr. Rogers explained how nightshade vegetables can stir up arthritis in some people: I immediately thought of Papa who smoked (tobacco is nightshade) and ate potatoes (another nightshade) every day of his life. He had severe rheumatoid arthritis. I wondered if this was the source of our woes.

I cut out the nightshades — potatoes, tomatoes, peppers (except black and white peppercorns, which are not in the same family), and eggplant. Fortunately, I have never smoked but my husband did for years and had quit again six months ago. I told him that going back was only an option if he wanted a divorce. Cigarettes or me — a dangerous choice to give any ex-smoker!

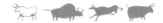

Eggplant has never appealed to me but all the others were very difficult because it meant no pizza, no lasagna, no French fries, no BLTs, no baked potatoes! How can you live in our society without pizza or fries?

The other thing about her book that impressed me right away was the information on minerals, especially magnesium. She shone a spotlight on the function of calcium and magnesium in the contraction and relaxation of muscles. With my muscles so tight, it was no wonder I needed massive doses of magnesium. She explained that the body attempts to keep up the blood level of magnesium. To do this, it takes magnesium from voluntary muscles and hence, muscles spasms. If there is still not enough, the body then turns to involuntary or smooth muscles such as organs like the heart. Perhaps this explained why I had been having up to twenty arrhythmias a minute. Arrhythmias are often described as 'skipped' heart beats when they are really an irregularity in rhythm with one beat coming too soon after another and then the longer gap until the next, feeling rather like hiccups in the chest. Uncomfortable! Maybe this also explained why the arrhythmias had decreased, since beginning the magnesium, from twenty a minute down to just a couple per minute.

Other symptoms of magnesium deficiency included neurological ones, such as anxiety and depression! Perhaps I wasn't a basket case after all. Just magnesium deficient. How come my magnesium test showed only a slightly low level but nothing dramatic? Again, Dr. Rogers' book explained. Since the body tries to keep the blood level up, the magnesium blood test can be deceiving.

My experience seemed to agree with this. I was taking over 800 mg of magnesium citrate in supplement form daily with no protest from my body. Diarrhea is the body's usual protest against too much magnesium. And I was getting 1000 mg in injections. Either I was terribly deficient or I wasn't absorbing it. I have since learned that there are people in both camps.

After reading Dr. Roger's book and doing the metabolic diet and the anti-yeast diet, I was all set to shift to a more vegetarian, macrobiotic sort of diet. I ordered Dr. Rogers recipe book, *Macro Mellow,* and embarked on a frenzy of cooking.

In one way, it was wonderful that I could even contemplate making some of the stuff. Peeling turnips had been an impossibility six months before. Cutting them generally still was — but I was making progress. I whomped up cauldrons of soup full of seaweed and assorted vegetables. Some of it was very good. The split pea soup reminded me of Popeye's spinach in its effect. One bowl full and you were zinging! The black bean and beet soup looked terrible. You expected something to jump out of it and grab you — but it tasted great.

The problem was that I wasn't feeling consistently very well. Some days were good. I tried to take a community college course with a friend but some weeks I couldn't make the class.

Once, just before my appointment in Toronto, I had dinner at a Chinese restaurant which swore it used no MSG. The next day, I did some cleaning with chlorine bleach. Hardly able to see straight for headache, I caught the train to Toronto. The trip was a nightmare, I was hurting so much. I managed to get on the correct subway but was confused, missed my stop, and had to backtrack. My face was hot but not with embarrassment.

About then I was reading *Hoffer's Laws of Natural Nutrition,* published by Quarry Press, who had released my poetry book, *My Underwear's Inside Out: The Care and Feeding of Young Poets.* Dr. Hoffer recommends a four-step program for improving your health. As he cautions, you should have a "medical check up from your doctor, especially if you suspect you are experiencing the symptoms of any disease. Anything you and your doctor find must be corrected. After that you should follow a procedure of improving your diet and

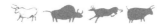

adding the correct supplements. It is desirable to do this with medical supervision, but you may find it very difficult to find a physician or nutritionist able to advise you. If you cannot find a physician, read everything you can about how to do so.

"To discover your optimum diet, I recommend the following 4 step program for pure health:

Step 1. Eliminate all the junk from your diet, especially all the free sugars, and any food you suspect you might be allergic to. Add vitamin C 1 gram after each meal. Stay on this diet for at least one month. If by then you feel well, this is your diet. If you are not any better or have gained only a little, examine your diet again for other possible food allergies, including allergies to dairy products and processed protein. Then eliminate them and carry on for another month. If you cannot find any other food allergies, go to step 2.

Step 2. Add a good vitamin B-complex tablet or one of the stress tablets. I like the B-complex 50 or 100 preparations. You can take as many as you wish but in most cases 1 to 3 tablets per day will be adequate. These all contain riboflavin or vitamin B-2, which will color the urine yellow. This is a good test whether or not the vitamins are being absorbed in the gastro-intestinal tract. Stay on this program for several months. If you have not reached the state of well being you want, then start to add other individual vitamins, minerals, and fatty acids. The main objective of this book is to describe these nutrients and how to use them well enough so that you can use them with safety. All these nutrients are compatible and can be taken together, usually with food in the stomach. Nutrients are compatible with all medication and with each other.

Step 3. For the rest of your life keep reviewing both your diet and the supplements you are taking because requirements

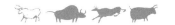

change with age, with sickness, with degree of stress. There is only one way of knowing and that is to be alert to the need to the changes in you and to the changes you must make in your diet. There is a constant need to maintain the adjustment between your needs and the food you eat.

Step 4. If you are still not well, you probably have very serious problems and will have to consult specialists in the field of orthomolecular medicine, the field of medicine I founded with such colleagues as Linus Pauling, Humphry Osmond, and Wilfrid and Evan Shute."

I was so happy to find a book that listed the steps Dr. M had put me through. Now if somebody asked about my treatment, I could tell them to get this book and read it. Mind you, the first step is enormous and requires reading in other books to navigate, but at least it's down in black and white.

I gave the book to Judy, a friend who was also going through this process, and she was equally excited. I called to congratulate my publisher on the release of Dr. Hoffer's book, and during the conversation, I came up with the idea of a reading group on the nutritional approach. After all, the books recommended by Dr. M had helped Judy and I, so why wouldn't they help others? Talking about the books had helped us even more.

At the doctor's office, I ran into a couple of ladies who were interested. The physiotherapist suggested someone. Judy and I hashed out a book list and a code of ethics. We set a date for a month hence to give the others time to find and read Dr. Hoffer's book. When we met, it was an explosion of discussion. Everyone found out something new. We started to take control of our own health and well-being — to take the bull by the horns.

Food Allergies

At our next appointment, Dr. M considered allergies. She suggested an allergy test — the ALCAT test. For testing a hundred items, it would cost me just about five hundred dollars and was a non-insured service. I gulped and said I would think about it. I thought it was at least worth a try figuring it out myself. How hard can allergies be to detect?

11/95 That day, it took me three tries to find the right entrance back onto the subway. When I finally made it to Union Station for the regular train to Kingston, my back was in terrible spasms. I asked the steward for some ice, put it in the self-sealing plastic bag I always carry, and applied it to the worst spot. Two miserable hours later, I was home. By bedtime, I was beginning to feel somewhat better, whether from the magnesium intravenous or just from the allergic reaction wearing off.

Already, I had cut the nightshade family out of my diet, but the results were not readily apparent. According to Dr. Rogers' book, it takes three months to break down the compounds this allergy creates in the body and thus three months to feel better.

After one month off nightshades, I had accidentally

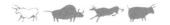

eaten some potato when we had a visitor for supper. I was so busy yakking that I dished up my dinner the same as the rest. Oops! Back to square one.

It was just as frustrating trying to eliminate other foods. I would cut one out for two weeks, try it again and still not be able to tell whether it was a problem or not. Some days I would feel reasonably well and other days I would feel rotten. There seemed to be no rhyme or reason. Beef, apples, wheat, milk, nothing seemed conclusive. By the end of November, I was ready to part with cash in exchange for any clues.

The allergy test was simple for me. Blood was taken and sent to the ALCAT lab in Florida. There the blood's conductivity was tested before exposure to allergens and again after each of the hundred items. Dr. M explained that the test was about 85 percent accurate so that it would be a place for us to start rather than the whole story. I paid my money and awaited my results, still trying to sort out what made me feel well or ill.

At least I wasn't in the horrible condition of the year before. I had good days. I could usually walk. I could usually make supper. I was doing a little writing. I was helping the Injured Workers' Association by filling out their grant applications.

We went to Matthew's concert at McGill University, over three hours away, and stayed overnight. I was in miserable pain after supper and at the concert, but I was there to hear the music and the applause. Lovely.

Next morning, on the train home, I made the mistake of having orange juice. The pain was unbelievable. As arranged, I went straight from the train station to my family doctor who had just begun to give me the magnesium injections once a week. I went home to crash and by evening was feeling a lot better.

I gave up trying to do the college course. There were just too many evenings when I was too sick to attend classes or, if

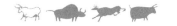

I did attend, something would make me sick, like perfume, magic markers, or just the air in the classroom.

Three days before Christmas, my holiday dinner was blown out of the water by the arrival of the ALCAT test results. Turkey, potatoes, corn, oranges, chocolate, broccoli, lettuce — all were a problem. So were beef, brewers yeast, cantaloupe, and four molds with unpronounceable names and unknown habitats. The one chemical allergy was a biggie — benzene which is in many petrochemical products, especially automobile exhaust. No wonder I hadn't been able to sort it all out.

For Christmas dinner, I had chicken, squash, turnips, and peas, with a poached pear for dessert. No wine. No cheese and crackers. No plum pudding. Remember — I still had the anti-yeast diet to observe as well. No treats, but it was the first Christmas in six years that I felt well enough to enjoy.

I also clued in that two of my supplements were probably doing me in. Cod liver oil! I turned out to be sensitive to cod. Vitamin C with bioflavonoids and rutin! The latter ingredients come from grapefruit rind and I am sensitive to citrus. I don't know whether to use the word 'allergic' or the word 'sensitive.' All I know is that some foods give me problems of various kinds from a bit of runny nose to gas pains to diarrhea to migraine-like headache and back spasms. The symptoms can last from a few minutes to many hours.

Besides giving eye-opening information about magnesium deficiency, Dr. Rogers' book, *Wellness Against All Odds*, describes the "macrobiotic diet" and its amazing ability to help people heal. A macrobiotic diet emphasizes whole grains (50 percent), beans (10 percent), local and sea vegetables (25 percent), seeds, local nuts, and seasonal fruits, prepared by stir frying, steaming, or boiling, though other foods and processes can be used if they are kept in balance according to the macrobiotic principles of yin and yang. As I said, I also ordered and received her cookbook, *Macro*

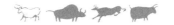

Mellow, which gives lots of recipes and tips on how to proceed. I needed to find alternatives to some of my allergic foods.

I read all about unfamiliar grains such as amaranth, quinoa, millet and buckwheat. I made the ultimate effort and went downtown to the largest health food store, returning with bags of these exotic seeds. The millet was reasonably easy to make into hot cereal for breakfast. It boiled up in a bearable twenty minutes or half an hour. With strawberries, it made a passable breakfast. The amaranth and quinoa (keen-wa) were a different story. It took nearly an hour of cooking before they were anywhere near edible. Their strong taste required something to make them appealing to my unaccustomed palate, and since my diet did not allow sugar, maple syrup, or honey, it had to be fruit. No milk. I was trying to cut out dairy products which are a common allergen.

But cooking time wasn't the main reason that the little bags of seeds disappeared from my refrigerator and freezer into the hoppers of our bird feeders, there to puzzle the chickadees. No, it was the allergy test that cleared up the mystery of why the different grains didn't make me feel very well. And closed — no, slammed — the door on the macrobiotic diet. When I went to my next appointment, Dr. M gave me a chart of molds and their usual habitats. I was allergic to the mold that can grow on grains! No wonder I was having inconsistent results. Sometimes the grains would have mold, sometimes not. There is no way to tell just by looking. And the kicker is that organic grains could have the most mold!

Per instructions, I got out the bottle of hydrogen peroxide from the bathroom cabinet, put a little in a clear glass, dropped in a few grains and watched for bubbles. Bubbles show that there is mold on the grain. That's when all the little bags of seed went out to the bird feeder, especially the organically-grown, expensive cream of wheat. On most people, the mold has no effect. For me, it's pronounced.

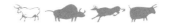

An incident soon after diagnosis made it quite clear. I made a berry cobbler for supper one Friday night when all the men were home. It smelled so good, I couldn't resist a spoonful.

Within half an hour, the left side of my back from my butt to my ear had started to spasm. My head ached on the left in migraine style. I felt awful — for several hours. I spent most of the night icing down the spasms. By morning it was mostly gone, except for a little residual tenderness.

The flour I had used was some that Matt had brought back from his university apartment. I tested it; the foam was profuse. This meant that grains or grain products were out unless I could test them for mold and they were clean. No crackers! No bread! No cereal! How would I survive?

Fortunately, the new bakery, where I had been buying sourdough breads of various kinds, had very high standards. Fresh flour every two weeks. I cautiously tried it out and, to my relief, no reaction occurred. This gave me grains for three days a week — whole-wheat, spelt/kamut, and rye.

The fourth day, I wanted to use rice. I bought some brown rice from the grocery. Anxiously, I tested it with peroxide. No luck, it fizzed up. I bought some organically-grown rice from the health food store. It was twice as expensive and even moldier. We had a box of Uncle Ben's Brown Rice® in the cupboard, so I decided to give that a try, in desperation. No reaction! It was fine. So now I had four grains for the four days of my new 'rotary' diet.

The Rotary Diet

To summarize the diet strategies. First, last June, I had eliminated sugar, yeast, and additives from my diet. Then, in the fall, I had eliminated the nightshades — potatoes, tomatoes, peppers, and eggplant.

With the results of the allergy test, I had a whole lot more to avoid — beef and turkey, lettuce and broccoli, oranges and chocolate, almonds and apples, corn and carob, cantaloupe and brewers yeast. (That's why alcohol in any form had always made me feel so rotten. I could never understand why people drank.)

But the suggested 'rotary' diet that came with my test results was incompatible with the sugar-free, yeast-free diet. I might starve! At the library, I was lucky enough to find *The Allergy Self-Help Book*. It gave a botanical breakdown of the food families and a good overview of the rotary diet. The whole idea is that a food or food family eaten on one day cannot be eaten again until 72 hours have passed. That time interval allows your body to clear that substance and any antibodies you might make to it.

So, I had to divide the foods I had left into menus for four days — making sure that each day would have enough calories, a green vegetable, a yellow vegetable, carbohydrates, proteins, and fats. Doris Rapp's excellent book, *Is This Your Child*, which I read a few months later, describes the diet I

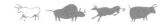

was trying to construct as "an impossible challenge." I'm glad I didn't know that at the time. I did realize that it was a tough one, especially first thing in the morning. All through January, I would wake up in a panic. "What am I going to eat today?" "Do we have any?" "Where can I get it?" "How will I cook it?"

I am fortunate in having a husband who will eat anything but tripe. As if my cooking is ever tripe! However, my son was a different story. He looked askance at dinner and said he would cook his own.

Here is the rotation I eventually worked out:

Day One: peas, carrots, celery, parsnips, parsley (the parsley family), rice, chicken, eggs, ginger, bananas, echinacea tea.

Day Two: cabbage, kale, Brussels sprouts, radishes, turnip, cauliflower, rutabagas (the cabbage family), tuna, rye, peaches, plums, nectarines, clove tea.

Day Three: lentils, beans, squash, cucumber, lamb, berries, spelt and kamut, garlic, raspberry leaf tea.

Day Four: spinach, beets, chard, sweet potatoes, asparagus, salmon, kiwi fruit, whole wheat, dill, mint tea.

That was it. Just barely enough foods to go around. Day Two wasn't very appetizing and Day Four didn't have much variety but there just wasn't anything else left. I could vary the fish a bit as long as I avoided the cod/haddock family. Even so, I didn't have enough oils to rotate. Olive oil and butter were it. Corn was out. I soon found that safflower and canola were related to the composite (lettuce) family and made me feel worse.

That was the best thing about the rotary diet. I could tell very quickly what food agreed with me. Remember — the

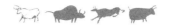

allergy test was only 85 percent accurate. I now had to test the assumptions. A pear, eaten for breakfast, made me feel weak, even though the allergy test had labeled it safe. Could it be the pesticides on the pear? I found out later that cooking tree fruits destroyed an enzyme that often causes allergic reactions. There is a cross allergy with birch pollen involved here.

Blueberries gave me terrible gas pains and diarrhea. Onions made my nose run and upset my stomach a bit. I kept trying to add yogurt but finally learned that allergic reactions damage the tips of the villi in the intestine so that they do not produce the enzyme needed to digest dairy products. It takes the villi two weeks to recover. I would have to wait until I was not having reactions to try dairy products again.

However, butter seemed to be all right, and so did olive oil. They became my stand-bys, with flax oil for salad dressings. Not enough to rotate but enough to sustain me. Later on I thought that the Shaklee® peanut butter was all right, giving me another oil source.

The rotary diet did not happen all at once. It took a month of experimentation, another month to learn how to shop — how much to buy, where to buy it. Another month to coordinate with my family's preferences. And so on. Occasionally the rotation would be superseded by a family event — birthday, anniversary, graduation, etc. I would eat what I could of foods safe for me and not worry. The next day would be time enough to go back to the rotation.

Occasionally a reliable food would act up. For example, one day a mango left me feeling weak, but when I thought about it, it was a new crop of mangoes from a different source than usual and the fruit had the tell-tale black marks left by gases used to speed ripening. I was probably reacting to the ripening agent. This happened another time with bananas. And this suggested to me, along with my allergy to benzene, that the environment might be a cause of some of my pain.

The Rotary Diet

Environmental Allergies

S o with the food situation somewhat stabilized, I turned my attention to my environment. Hah! That sounds so calm and organized. What actually happened was chaotic and crisis-provoking.

01/96 The ALCAT test results showed that besides multiple food problems, I was sensitive to some of the molds that can grow on rugs, paper, damp basements, etc. All of these we had 'up the hoop.'

The Allergy Self-Help Book (unfortunately no longer in print but there are other useful books like Doris Rapp's *Is This Your Child* and *Tired or Toxic* by Dr. Rogers) recommended decontaminating the bedroom first. I persuaded my husband and son to take the carpet out. There was a bit of grumbling about cold feet on a bare bedroom floor, but I countered with slippers and beguiling promises of how much better I might feel. Talk about your sweet talk!

It was a cold, dark January evening — something like the beginning to one of Snoopy's novels — when Matt and Chris began. This is important for you to feel the proper sympathy in a few minutes. I hovered, watching. Then my face began to redden. My nose stuffed up and I became agitated. I had to get out! I called a friend and escaped. Actually, I made

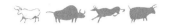

the rounds of a couple of friends — a refugee from my own home, driving around in the cold and dark. There now! I hope you feel properly sympathetic.

In a couple of hours, I called home. They were done. The carpet was rolled up and left in the living room.

"Please put it outside!" I couldn't even stand being in the room with it. What was I reacting to in that carpet? Was it mold, dust, dust mites, or what?

While Matt and Chris wrapped it in plastic and put it out on the deck, I washed the bedroom floor. Again my face reddened. By then I was too tired and sick to care. I fell into bed. In the morning, there was one bit of carpet left in the bedroom closet. Matthew went at and pulled it out. I followed up washing the floor. Again the red face.

"Mom, I think I can smell something in there. It smells like the flea spray."

He was right! Eight years ago, the house was sprayed for an outbreak of cat fleas. And the stuff still smelled after all that time! Maybe the chemical was a clue to my problems. I began to think about chemicals as well as molds. After all, the ALCAT test had shown an allergy to benzene — an element of gasoline and other petrochemicals.

The men next tackled the carpet in Matt's room, but there was no tile underneath. We bought some parquet and the best non-volatile glue we could find. Even then, with the door closed and the windows open to the February air, I felt sick from the fumes. Despite that, in the next few days, I took everything out of my bedroom closet and disposed of armloads of old stuff. Anything with a musty smell was washed or tossed, depending on the possibilities.

I washed all the bedding. I vacuumed the vertical blinds. I mopped down the walls. Hey! I can't do stuff like that! Well, I can if I spend all night on ice packs and cram six magnesium capsules a day into myself, have a magnesium IV once a week, take 30 other supplements a day, rest 25 times,

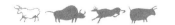

and have someone cook dinner when I collapse. Still, it was encouraging to be able to do something to help.

The basement — oh dreaded word — was next. Half the basement floor had wooden subfloor with carpet. Musty to the nth degree. Crowbar at the ready, Chris attacked. Plywood flew. The pile of old carpet grew outside in the carport. We had to decide what to put down in its place. Something that wouldn't rot, something that wouldn't outgas chemicals. Hopefully, please, something we could afford. We found a deal on ceramic tiles and went with the most environmentally-friendly glue we could find. It was beautiful, didn't smell, and we couldn't afford not to put it down. Professionals had it done in a couple of days.

All would have gone smoothly if someone hadn't dropped a rag in the laundry tub, so that when I put on a wash, the tub overflowed. Everything piled in the old half of the basement (with vinyl flooring) was now standing in a puddle. I had a fit. Chris and Matt had a fit too and then went to work mopping and drying. The humidity level and the mold level rose. Ah me, solve one problem and another arises to take its place. The Hydra of mythology with a myriad heads.

Some of the living room and dining room carpets had to stay because there was only subfloor under certain areas and we couldn't figure out what to put down that I could tolerate. Even wooden flooring was out because I couldn't handle the fumes from whatever was used to finish it. That problem would just have to hang fire.

In the living room, I have a comfy glider rocker that I like a lot. For some unknown reason, I had stopped sitting in it. Instead, I would head for the sofa on the other side of the room. Even when I would consciously decide to sit in that chair, I would fidget and soon move. I began to wonder if the large, potted schefflera beside the chair was the problem. Initially, Chris rebelled at the idea of losing plants. In February, in Ontario, there isn't much greenery besides the

outside evergreenery. Chris enjoyed the plants. Besides, the two big scheffleras had been anniversary presents a few years ago.

I persuaded. "Just lift up the plastic pot so we can check out the wooden tub." He gave in. The wooden tub was black with mold. So was the matching one in the dining room. There was no denying that the black sooty coating smelled like Dracula's coffin. I watched, with a sad but determined face, while Chris, with a sad but determined face, carted the two big trees out to the frozen compost heap and certain death. Even more, my late father had made the wooden tubs for me years ago and I did not like to put them out in the snow with the carpet. But there seemed to be no choice.

It seemed that everything was being taken away — food, clothing, cheery decor, plants, our cash reserve. We only hoped but didn't know for sure that the effort would pay off.

The glider rocker again became my favorite chair.

What could cause a person to become so allergic in middle life? This problem is fodder for biochemistry for the next few decades. It's not simple or one-sided. I had been reading *The Canary and Chronic Fatigue* by Dr. Majid Ali. He also believes that we can run out of nutrients to deal with the chemicals in our environments. There is only so much each person's body can do. 'Oxidative injury' is his term for the problem.

In *The E.I. Syndrome*, Dr. Sherry Rogers explains that the chemicals can damage the T-suppresser cells which mediate the amount of antibodies you produce to foods. Damaged cells can produce far too much. Hence, the overload of antibodies to things which should not provoke them.

In *Tired or Toxic*, she explains that magnesium is required in over 300 reactions in the body, including those that help remove toxic chemicals. If you are deficient in magnesium, the detoxification reactions become backlogged. The chemicals are not processed but remain in your system.

When Dr. M gave me a list of the clinical signs of magnesium deficiency, I found myself in many places. The bone spurs I suffered on my heels in my twenties were probably due to magnesium deficiency because calcium deposited in inappropriate places is one symptom. My difficulty with anesthetics after every surgery indicated an inability to process chemicals. The subsequent muscle spasms perhaps showed that my body was struggling to find enough magnesium. The Morton's neuroma could have been due to calcium deposits irritating the nerve in my foot. The anxiety and the 'blues' that so often dogged me could also be a symptom of magnesium deficiency. Stress creates chemicals in the body which also require magnesium to break down. Fancy that! The arrhythmias in which my heart was 'skipping' up to twenty beats a minute were another sign.

As for chemical overload, the last year I taught included a lot. We had the house sprayed for cat fleas. There was the head lice epidemic — I used the toxic shampoo twice. My junior kindergarten room had a new carpet glued down and new laminated furniture. In the oven in that classroom, the parents had stored, for lack of space anywhere else, the margarine tubs they used for relish on hot dog day. I turned on the oven to bake a craft project and the tubs burned, producing a dioxin-laden smoke. When I moved to a different school, it was promptly painted. The furnace at home was found to have a cracked heat exchanger which could have been leaking carbon monoxide. I even had a new car with all its smells. Top these off with a magnesium-depleting medication prescribed for my back problem, amitriptyline (a.k.a. Elavil®.) Plus, the sicker I became, the less energy I had to prepare good meals.

I could have died from a stroke, brought on by the magnesium deficiency, or the pain and depression could have driven me to suicide. Which brings me to another part of my medical history. Maybe my mother didn't have encephalitis

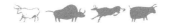

but an undiagnosed case of the same problem as mine. She had a car accident, a kidney problem, pain, anxiety, and finally depression leading to suicide. Dr. M thinks it is more than likely that she had a similar condition to my own. The tragedy that has shadowed my life makes more sense.

So here I am stuffing in magnesium citrate capsules, up to six x 140 mg a day, plus a multimineral which adds another 180 mg. Add to that magnesium sulfate by injection once a week. If you take too much magnesium you can reliably tell because you will have diarrhea. I had no such problem.

Dr. M had recommended the injections from the beginning, but I wasn't sure, and my family doctor was even less so. For six months, we had waffled. I would have one injection a month at Dr. M's, but that obviously wasn't enough since the effect wore off within a day or so. However, my family doctor could see that I was making progress, and when I went to Montreal for my son's graduation recital, he agreed to give me the magnesium on my return. The injection brought such relief! I walked out a different person.

Then began the weekly injections that were to continue for over a year. They helped me, finally, to rid myself of the amitriptyline which I had been cutting back slowly for six months. By Christmas 1996, I was free of it. At last, my brain could belong to me again. Delightful to be free of the fog the medication caused. Of course, that was about the time the allergy message got through and I had to start the rotary diet and the environmental changes. It was a good thing I had more of my brain to do them.

Sauna Depuration

There were still several flies in the ointment — all those chemicals to detoxify. The theory is that the adipose (fatty) tissues store toxins. So as I lost fat, thirty pounds over eight months, the toxins were released into my system. Some could be processed but a lot were undoubtedly redeposited. It is difficult to flush them out. What to do?

03/96 Dr. M gave me some medical journal articles on a procedure known as sauna depuration. According to the research, this procedure helps people rid themselves of toxic chemicals stored in the adipose tissue. Because of my symptoms, my history, and the process of elimination we had been using for the past year, chemical overload would seem to be a safe bet as the cause of some of my problems.

It is possible to mobilize the fat using niacin, but then the body must be able to process the released chemicals. Since my detoxification system wasn't working well because of the magnesium deficiency, they would just settle back into my tissues, more concentrated than before. This might explain why, as I lost the weight, I went through periods of feeling miserable.

I read the articles. First, the protocol called for aerobic

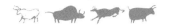

exercise such as running, swimming, or cycling. The purpose is to increase the heart rate and start the sweating. For me, the most aerobic thing I could do was walk and that not very quickly. Pushing for faster has always led to problems. What could I do?

The next step is to take the niacin in gradually increasing doses over the three weeks of the treatment. The niacin increases sweating and mobilizes the fat. The third step is to go into the sauna, at lower temperatures, for increasing amounts of time, with breaks for showers, fluids, vitamins, and minerals to prevent dehydration and food oils to replace the fat.

Chris read through the information and pointed out that I couldn't do *anything* for five hours a day, let alone exercise and sauna. My physiotherapist and family doctor pointed out the same thing. But I'm, to put it politely, determined as a terrier. My childhood pet actually was a Jack Russell terrier, so put it down to that. I kept thinking about Dr. M's accounts of other patients who could hardly walk the first day of the program and could jog by the end of it. I wanted to be the same. Three weeks of treatment seemed like nothing compared to the torture of the past seven years.

I called the institute providing the sauna depuration program to arrange things as quickly as possible. I had just a month before my few author readings would begin. I was most worried about my food. I would need somewhere to stay with kitchen facilities so I could prepare my rotary diet. I bought cans of chicken, tuna, salmon and other fish, a box of my safe rice, bags of beans and lentils, fruit and vegetables. How long can three weeks be? Just get through it one day at a time.

I took off for Toronto in great excitement — my car piled high — not many clothes but lots of food, books, etc. This was an adventure — something quite lacking in my usual regimen.

Sauna Depuration

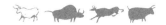

Traffic fumes bothered me, but I arrived in good time and was escorted to the home of a friend of the director where a room had been arranged. The room was pleasant enough, but it was in a basement. The director showed me around since the owners were out. She helped me unload the car and left. I felt agitated. I gathered up stuff for supper and went up to the kitchen to prepare it. As I cooked the Brussels sprouts and cauliflower, I began to feel quite peculiar. My vision began to change. My face felt hot. It was getting difficult to breathe. By the time dinner was ready, I knew I was having an allergic response to the house. What to do? I had to get out.

I tried to look up hotels in the phone book but my eyes wouldn't focus. I called a friend whose number I knew and asked him where the nearest hotel might be. He gave me a couple of options. I knew how to get to one of them. Somehow I flung everything back into the car, tidied the kitchen, and even left the porch light on and a note for my would-be hosts. How can you tell someone nicely that you are allergic to her house? Miss Manners hasn't carried that one lately.

The hotel wasn't much better — scented cleaning materials — but my symptoms subsided a bit. I went to a milk store for baking soda to see if that would help.

It was not a restful night. The polyester sheets felt burning hot. I wrapped my legs and feet in the cotton towels and used my own precious pillow from home.

The next morning, I breakfasted on a banana and the bread I had brought from home and hurried over to the institute to explain the problem. We spent the morning trying to find a place to stay that was in the affordable range and possible from an allergy point of view. No luck.

After lunch, I was scheduled to have various assessments. One was an interview. Another was a session of written tests. The Institute deals largely with substance abusers so personal history, habits, and psychology are important. Testing before and after treatment helps highlight the changes produced.

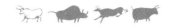

Sitting in their spare office, writing the tests, my back gradually began to seize up. I attributed it to hunching over the desk for an hour. After the test, I was in a lot of pain so the trainer and the director kindly offered to treat my back, as they were quite experienced in unknotting muscles.

I lay face down on the cot and they did their best. It didn't help. In fact, I felt worse. I wanted to get outside for some fresh air, so I walked to the corner, in the cold drizzle, for a newspaper. With still no place to stay, we decided I could use the spare office and perhaps it would do for the duration since there was a kitchen and shower downstairs. I unloaded my stuff from the car and set up camp in the office.

I headed downstairs to make my supper of salmon and sweet potato. The sauna room was also downstairs. The cedar smelled lovely. The director had suggested, half in jest, that I could always sleep in the sauna room. When I went back upstairs to my office-cum-bedroom and tried to go in, I realized what the problem was. There was an over-whelming (at least to me) smell of pesticide. I could barely go in long enough, holding my breath, to lug my stuff out in the hall! The cot mattress particularly exuded a miasma of the stuff! No wonder it made me feel sick!

I called my friends again. They had absolutely nowhere to put me since their small house was already bursting with themselves, their daughter, son-in-law, grandchild, and large dog. However, they had a futon mattress, brought it over and put it in the sauna room for me. They helped me take my bedding next door and put it through the laundromat since it all smelled of the pesticide. My friends left me reluc-tantly. I was beginning to be quite frightened and ill as well as tired out. I tried to get to sleep in the sauna but *something* was getting to me. My vision was going again and my face was getting hot.

I went into the office next to the sauna to call the director. She told me to take a taxi to her place. I stuffed my bedding, a

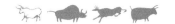

change of clothes, and my breakfast foods into a garbage bag and called a taxi. By 11:30, halfway across the city, exhausted but no longer reacting, I was ensconced on her living room sofa. I managed five hours of sleep.

The next morning was my pre-sauna-treatment check-up with Dr. M. After that another round of trying to find accommodation. I treated myself to a hot meal of plain chicken and carrots at a restaurant.

Back at the institute, they had been busy. It turned out that some Raid® had been sprayed downstairs in the kitchen area. Also there had been a minor flood and one washroom had a mold problem. The cot mattress had been fumigated some time in the past. They had thrown it out and scrubbed everything. I was breathing easier, but they decided I'd better try a sample of the blended oils (peanut, walnut, safflower and soy) they used as a supplement. I took a teaspoon full and in half an hour had a red face.

Time to head for home. This was definitely not going to work. Three hours of driving later — taking extra care because of my condition — I fell thankfully into my own blessed bed. I wasn't giving up on the sauna idea but it was definitely going to the back burner for a while.

The anniversary of my first visit to Dr. M came and went. I was still having a magnesium sulfate injection once a week but something was happening. The day of my shot, I couldn't sleep properly. I would wake up way too early and then couldn't get back to sleep.

The next week, the night of my shot, for some reason, I reached for the calcium tablets at bedtime. Always before, calcium had kept me awake. This time I slept. The next week, I needed calcium for two nights after the injection. The following week, the calcium didn't work at all. I was feeling peculiar and rather frantic.

Then my family doctor went on holidays, and I didn't receive a shot for two weeks. That was fortuitous because I

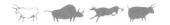

realized I didn't need it. In fact, my need for the oral supplement had decreased from six capsules a day to two.

Dr. M suggested that another mineral deficiency was being unmasked. Potassium was a strong possibility, but maybe something else. I went home wondering. For two more weeks, I kept waking up too soon. That is how some of this book was written. Then, I thought to go back to my original blood tests. Bingo! Low calcium! I tried the calcium again with my bedtime magnesium. It helped a little. Not enough. My husband offered me one of his Cal/Mag supplements which contained 300 mg of each as opposed to the 250/140 I had tried. That night I slept straight through for the first time in a month. Delightful!

This reinforced to me that reevaluating the supplements is a constant process.

I have had to continue to reevaluate the supplements constantly. If I am accidentally exposed to more chemicals than I can handle, I have to take more vitamin C and more magnesium. With the sauna and other detoxification procedures, I have to be very careful of my electrolytes, especially potassium. With my hormonal cycle, I need more evening primrose oil to sleep properly at the middle and end of the month. It seems never to be simple. With time, my need for and dependence on supplements should decrease, according to the experts.

Parasites

D r. M had another 'suggestion' — the quiet word that signals another horrendous upheaval. This time it was the bug connection. Many people have some sort of intestinal parasite. In Europe and many other parts of the world, an annual purge of the intestinal tract is the usual thing. The jury is out on whether the most common parasites cause health problems or not. Some, like Helen Kruger, feel that all our health problems can be traced to parasites. Traditional medicine scoffs at the notion. The patient is the tug-of-war rope in between. However, if you are not well, isn't it worth trying every avenue? Some people do not begin to recover until the parasite problem is cleared up. I know some like that.

07/96 That summer I dutifully submitted the samples again and was told I had a common St. Lawrence River valley parasite, blastocystus hominus. Since I am allergic to citrus, and thus, perhaps, the citricidal used against parasites, I decided to consult the nutritionist in town who does muscle testing. She tested me with the grapefruit seed extract and then with black walnut oil extract. The former was not good but the latter seemed quite strong. I decided to try it. Her advice was to start out very gradually with one drop three

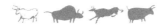

times a day and work my way up to the five drops.

The stuff tasted unpleasant. Black walnut trees actually kill whatever tries to grow under them, so black walnut oil extract is a fairly potent remedy. I followed instructions and on day four felt the runny nose and flu-like symptoms associated with die-off. I continued the treatment for another five days just to be sure. Acidophilus was, of course, part of the treatment to repopulate my intestinal flora.

When I was retested a month later, the bugs were reduced but some still remained. I had to do it all over again! Another book, *Allergies: Diseases in Disguise*, by Carolee Bateson-Koch, recommends a two-stage attack to interrupt the life cycle of the wee beasties. As frustrated as I was, I wasn't nearly as bothered as another friend who had to be tested at the Redpath Lab in Toronto, which found much more exotic creatures. The treatment was correspondingly unpleasant and much longer but ultimately successful. *Guess What Came to Dinner?* by Ann Louise Gittleman, was the book she read to understand the situation better, but I never did get up the nerve to read it with her. We all have our limitations. I'm sure I would if I needed it to progress.

I had done something in May that I had to forgo a year previously. The Sudbury Board of Education had invited me to visit and read to classes from my books. I decided that this year I could try. It was scary after my experience away in March, but I am nothing if not determined. 'Pig-headed' comes to mind. I flew there despite protests from the sponsoring organization who wanted me to take a cheaper route. No way was I ready to handle an eight-hour drive. A two-hour flight was almost more than I could take. My luggage was mostly food, a pile of supplements, a few clothes, and some books to sell.

I managed the four days quite well despite an allergic reaction to an episode of painting in the hotel bar, a reaction to one of the meals out, and more to perfume on some

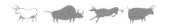

of the teachers. 'Quite well' means going to bed directly after supper, no sightseeing, coffee enemas daily, ice and heat on my back several times a night, and, for the first time in months, some painkillers. It was wonderful to be doing something *in addition to* health care.

It took a couple of weeks to recover and then I did an even stupider thing. I was feeling well and thinking about the sauna program. It was a nice day at the park where I was walking. I felt so buoyant that I decided to run a few steps. I did and it felt okay. Bad move. It took three weeks to recover from that escapade.

About that time we found a portable sauna for sale, but it could also be rented. With a friend also disabled with FM, I rented it for a month. Being cautious, for once in my life, or perhaps reluctant to mess up again so soon, we started with the lowest temperature for 20 minutes. We hardly sweated at all. We dutifully made sure to have our water and salty snacks. Over the month, we worked up to two 20-minute sessions at 145 degrees, three times a week. It did ease aching muscles quite a lot. For my friend, who was quite restricted in walking as well, it was the first time since her condition had become so severe that she could work up a sweat.

Then the month was up but we knew a sauna was in our future. We went out and ordered sauna kits with promises from Matt that he would assemble them. In a month, they arrived and Matthew went to work tearing up a corner of the basement and fitting in the sauna. The wood was sorted out on the floor. It smelled so clean and fresh. At last, something that smelled good to me. I should have checked the portents for that day.

The sound of disaster was the sound of water — water overflowing the laundry tubs and flooding the vinyl flooring where the sauna wood was sitting! Someone who shall remain nameless — actually Michael — had carefully placed the rag he had used to wash the floor over the edge of the

laundry tub to dry. The vibration of the washer, transmitted to the laundry tubs, had caused the rag to fall into the tub and block the drain. Once more, the humidity level, the frustration level, and the activity level went up in sync. The only good thing was that the wood was piled on the cardboard in which it had been shipped. Chris managed to move most of it and 'wet vac' the water so that only a few pieces were dampened a touch.

I didn't discover the rest of the problem until a couple of days later when I was sweeping up some of the sawdust and shavings where Matt was working. I thought the dust was bothering me. My nose began to run and I didn't want to breathe.The corner where the sauna was going had supported a bookcase which had been dismantled and the books piled, I thought, on boards. *Most* of the books were on boards. A few dozen were not! And they were in a rare old state of green fuzzy. Chris once again bagged books, and sadly, as they were some of his sci-fi books, tossed them in the garbage. Such sacrifices this process has entailed, though any process you care to name seems to require them.

Then there was the wiring contretemps with our neighbor giving directions that fried some wires and with Chris breaking the new temperature control knob. "How should I know that just dropping it would break it!" Our neighbor also had a vicious cold which promptly colonized the rest of us as well. For three weeks I didn't care what else happened.

The sun finally came out. It really had rained non-stop that month! Everything was now dry! I felt better and I started to use the sauna. I tried the previously-successful strategy of 20 minutes in, cool off with a glass of water and then 20 minutes again. This time there was a problem. Five minutes into the second session I began to feel claustrophobic and anxious. I couldn't make myself stay there. I had to get out.

Dr. M to the rescue. "Salts," she said. "Your electrolytes are out of balance. Take a glass of water with a teaspoon of

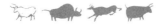

sea salt dissolved in it and when you feel like that, drink some. And get that potassium!" I got the potassium, made up my glass of sea salt water and tried it. It worked. I could now handle a half hour and then another 20 minutes, no problem.

Rereading the journal article on sauna depuration, I noticed the remarks on oil supplementation. That was the next thing to control. Now, on my break, dripping sweat and looking as lovely as a drowned cat, I would drink the salty water and have a snack with either peanut butter or olive oil on a piece of bread.

I was afraid to try the niacin without further consultation. However, I was taking two B50 complex tablets every day anyway and they contain 100 mg of niacin. Not a lot, but something.

Osteopathy

About this time there appeared a popular book about alternative medical methods, Andrew Weil's *Spontaneous Healing*. In that book, there was a chapter that struck a chord with me. The chapter describes the work of an old-fashioned osteopath.

Osteopaths go back to 1874 in the United States and have training considered the equivalent to that of M.D.s. However, originally, the focus was quite different. The smooth functioning of the body's structure — the bones and muscles allowing the organs to do their work unimpeded.

What interested me in the book was the discussion of places that are 'snagged' or 'jammed' in the body and the treatments to release those places. That's exactly how my body felt. I kept envisioning my back muscles as a spider web with the webbing snagged in places. In many acute episodes, my spine felt jammed at some point or other. In addition, the description of the restrictions in breathing sounded familiar too. In fact, the breathing problem had sent me to the doctor long before all this began. It all seemed to make sense.

I was also interested in the importance placed on incidents when the wind was knocked out of you, or when there was a blow to the head or a fall on the tailbone. The wind was knocked out of me quite a few times as a child, and I

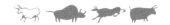

had knocks to various parts and the usual quotient of falls as an adult.

The only problem was that osteopaths are as rare as hen's teeth in Ontario. The nearest one was in Montreal, over 300 kilometers away. There was one other avenue to explore: some physical therapists are trained in one aspect of osteopathy — cranial-sacral treatment. I phoned around to find out if there was anyone in the area with that training. Some chiropractors do the work, but I was reluctant to have any aggressive chiropractic manipulation in the bargain.

I told my physiotherapist I was interested in trying the therapy and asked if he knew anyone he could safely recommend. He suggested a clinic, and so I made an appointment. I went for an assessment, which consisted of the usual range-of-motion examination and then the unfamiliar — extremely gentle probing of sacrum, head, and neck. She commented on restrictions and thought treatment would help.

At that moment, our extended health carrier decided my file should be reviewed, and physiotherapy was stopped pending their approval. By the time we had fought that battle and coverage was reinstated, I was embroiled in the sauna affair and had nothing left over to investigate new therapies.

08/96 I did go back a few months later to find a different therapist, Miriam, and — oh joy — she was studying osteopathic strategies at the newly-instituted College of Osteopathy in Toronto. The time was obviously right.

She was very interested in the rest of my program. She felt that there was much more chance for success with the support of the nutritional therapies. When I told her about the reading groups I had organized for exploration and discussion of nutritional problems and therapies, she was so interested she asked me to set one up for her patients, which I did.

Osteopathy

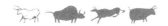

The first few sessions with Miriam were the same kind of gentle pressure on sacrum, head, and neck. Cranial-sacral therapists can feel a pulse different than the cardiac one — a pulse in the spinal fluid. The pressure aims to decompact joints and allow this pulse to beat freely. Blows or injuries to the head or spinal column can interfere with this pulse. Again, a history is required — a history of blows and injuries quite different from the history required for other specialties. I trotted out my car accident, the blow to my head from a falling portable blackboard, the surgeries, the baseball that knocked me down, and all the times I knocked the breath out of myself as a child.

I felt some interesting effects. One was the solving of the "stuffy nose" mystery. For years, I have had a stuffy nose but it is a very selective stuffy nose. If I lie on one side in bed, then that side may be stuffy, but the stuffiness can disappear instantly or shift suddenly from one side to the other. With the cranial-sacral manipulation, it became quite clear that the stuffy nose had something to do with my neck and my trigeminal nerve. When something in my neck impinged on the nerve, it could cause the stuffy nose and just as suddenly clear it up when released. This went also for the "mystery cough" which had annoyed me so unpredictably for the last few years. This does not explain, however, what causes the neck to get out of whack and impinge on the nerve or what causes the nerve to be so reactive.

After some treatments, I would have a miserable night while everything readjusted to new positions. One night I felt as if I had to constantly swallow. Another night I coughed. Another night I couldn't breathe very well. Everything finally relented and calmed down. One day while out for a walk, my husband pointed to a bird in a tree. I looked way, way up searching for the bird and induced a splendid coughing fit. As soon as I looked down again, the coughing subsided! Another night, I used the strain-counter strain technique on

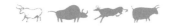

my own face — finding a trigger point and gently urging it in the direction that didn't hurt. I relieved the stuffy nose greatly. Of course, it depends on how tight my muscles are, and thus on my magnesium status, whether I have much success or not.

The other end went through some adjustments, too. The sacral manipulations would cause my digestive system to gurgle to life, and I would have unaccustomed loose bowels. The work on my neck also caused a decrease in my pulse rate of about ten points.

Another day Miriam asked me to lie on my stomach and began to press down in places, starting with my shoulders. It had been so long since anyone had touched my back that I had forgotten why I didn't let anyone near it. Suddenly she hit a spot mid-back and my arms and legs flew out and I yelled.

"Aah!" she said. "Original sin!"

It took me two weeks to recover. Almost record time for me.

"Can't stretch those muscles at all," she said. "We'll have to try strain-counterstrain." She would locate a trigger point, press on it, and then assist me to subtly change position until the point ceased to hurt. She would keep the pressure on and follow the muscle as it twitched and shifted until it would finally relax. Miriam started out cautiously, not wanting to "blow me up." I was quite happy not to be "blown up." She warned me I might feel some effects from releasing the trigger points.

There is a lot of debate as to what material is actually in the trigger points. Some, like Devin Starlanyl, who wrote *Fibromyalgia and Myofascial Pain Syndrome*, say calcium phosphate. Most agree that whatever it is, releasing it into the system may make a person feel unpleasant for a bit. At least I had a lot of the detoxification strategies in place — extra magnesium, skin brushing, sea salt and soda baths, coffee enemas and the sauna. For the trigger points furthest from

the injury site, these kept the effect down to a few hours of discomfort. The discomfort was not muscle spasm or pain. It was soreness and a general feeling of malaise, like a mild case of flu. The trigger point itself did not spasm. After the treatment, it felt 'unsnagged.' I felt as though I could move more freely. I began to be able to breathe better. I began to be able to sing again and surprised myself that I could sing more in tune than I had thought I could. Obviously, it wasn't just my ear that was at fault in my previously out-of-tune efforts. My ability to breathe properly and control my breathing had a great deal to do with it.

Then there was the day Miriam decided to tackle one of the points in the serratus posterior. This was the muscle with the most problems — the one that caused me the most grief. She spent a lot of the session on that one point, but wasn't quite satisfied that it had totally released. It hadn't and it caused havoc. A nerve was trapped and I spent the next two days with ice packs and extra magnesium trying to ease the pain.

She released it in a few moments in the next session and spent the rest of the time on another trigger point, one of the "bad guys," as she termed it. It bucked and sidestepped like a wild horse. When the first layer finally relaxed, the layer underneath took over. It would seem to finish but then resume its activities. When it finally seemed played out, Miriam's finger was hot. I expected to experience quite an effect from this, but the rest of the day went well as I 'ran' errands and went for a walk. I took the precaution of a coffee enema during the day.

That night I didn't sleep very well, waking up after every couple of hours. About five a.m., I gave up and went downstairs for a sauna. As the day wore on, I felt increasingly miserable. About noon a headache started niggling at me. I wasn't sure what type it was, although it was over the top of my head and into my sinuses. Could it be a cold coming on? Chris had

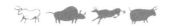

one. By supper time, the headache was bigger, so I tried ice, which didn't do anything. I had a sea salt and soda bath which helped enough that I fell asleep. Two hours later, I was awake with the headache again, so I tried heat, ice, and an Alka Seltzer Gold in case it was an allergic reaction. Alka Seltzer Gold contains no painkillers, just sodium bicarbonate. This electrolyte solution counters the effect of allergic reactions which tend to disrupt the body's PH balance. A teaspoon of baking soda in water is a less effective alternative. Many other commercially available electrolyte drinks have ingredients which may be allergens themselves, such as orange juice, sugar, and preservatives.

After half an hour the headache was just as bad, if not worse, so I knew then that it was toxicity from the work on the trigger point. Although I didn't especially want to go through the whole rigmarole at 2:00 a.m., I went through a coffee enema. In half an hour, the headache was gone. Thank you, Sherry Rogers. I got back to sleep. Waking two hours later in a lather of sweat, I got up and went to the kitchen, but by the time I got there I was feeling quite faint. Perhaps the detoxification procedures had thrown my electrolytes out again. I took some potassium and curled up with a book to see if it would pass. And it did. Back to sleep again.

The next day I felt somewhat ill and took extra supplements of the minerals, lots of water, and didn't do much — a sea salt and soda bath in the morning and a sauna at night. By the next day at noon, I was perking up and I don't mean coffee. I may never be able to actually drink coffee again. However, my back was feeling quite fine. The previously-trapped nerves were no longer causing any twitching or spasms.

Miriam had some observations on my experience. One was that before her osteopathic training she would have considered that she had just done too much with me. Another was that without my detoxification procedures, it would have been much more difficult and prolonged getting through

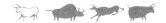

the aftermath of the work on the trigger point.

My observation was that there were more of these nasty spots to do, and I was not looking forward to working through them one bit. I was looking forward only to being finished with them and feeling freedom in my back instead of the miserable restrictions that had hobbled me for so long. We had been working for four months and had three more months left on the insurance meter.

There were several more nasty points that caused similar reactions. Having my magnesium shot the same day in a couple of instances reduced the misery significantly. Later on, the points caused much less problem. I could still tell that I was going through the process but it was much less intense.

The pay-off was that, as each point was done, my back was less restricted. On good days, usually a couple of days before a new point was to be done, I could do things I hadn't been able to do in years. I could clean the bathrooms. I'm sure everyone has that as a supreme goal! I could dust a room, maybe two rooms. I could clean out the refrigerator. If only I could consume some of the things in there! I could clean a closet. And I could do it without requiring ice packs and heat packs and pain killers and TENS® and muscle relaxants and acupuncture!

The best of all was the night in January 1997 when I went to a movie — something I hadn't done in a couple of years because the pain was just not worth it. My library reading group had selected *The English Patient* since the movie had just been released. It was a long movie — two and a half hours — but I enjoyed it thoroughly. It was bliss to sit and not spend the whole time squirming in agony.

The ironic part was that the title character was a dying man who had been severely burned, whose breathing was difficult, and who could barely move. As he lay there making shallow little breaths, enduring both the indignity of having

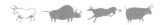

everything done for him as well as the pain, I found it simple to understand the psychology, to empathize. I felt so lucky to have another chance.

Besides dealing with the trigger points, osteopathy has strategies which can profoundly affect organ function. My original injury had been in my mid back and the muscles there had been tight for eight years. In the summer of '96, my DHEA level was found to be half what is normal for a woman of my age. DHEA is an adrenal hormone. I had tried a small amount of DHEA supplement, and it had picked up my energy levels quite a bit, but in November, my level was still only two-thirds normal.

What's this got to do with tight muscles in the mid back? The taut muscles were over the lower thoracic vertebrae whose nerves supply the adrenal gland. The kidneys and adrenal glands are directly under the muscles that were so tight. Therefore the blood supply had been compromised for eight years. Miriam decided I was ready for a strategy to loosen up that area. She did it and I was quite sore and stiff for a few days. I developed some other mysterious symptoms, such as flushing and sweating a few times. I began to sleep less well, waking up several times a night. I was restless by day as well.

I had my family doctor check my DHEA level. The test came back normal! I immediately stopped taking the supplement. Unfortunately, with the stress on my system from so many allergic reactions and so much detoxification work, the level went down again and perhaps I should have tapered off the supplement more slowly. We shall try again.

One of the last bad snow storms of February turned out to be a blessing in disguise. It was a day when I was scheduled for physiotherapy and I was taking a friend for her appointment as well. By the time I had to leave in the morning, the fellow who plows our driveway had still not appeared. Chris had managed to get out for work and so I thought I would

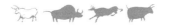

give it a shot too. I made it as far as the turnaround, backed and was ready to start hood first to the road. With the drift, the highway plow's deposit and the underlying ice from an earlier thaw, I didn't make it.

I had to walk back to the house (a hundred feet) through the snow to roust Matthew from bed. I got a partial bag of kitty litter from the basement to put on the icy bits and walked back down to the car. Matt came and, with the help of a passerby, managed to release the car. Off I went, picked up my friend and had my physiotherapy. Unfortunately, the drive wasn't plowed when I arrived home either. I made it half way. Another slog up the driveway to call for help. When the plow arrived I bundled up and slogged back down to drive while the man shoveled and did the necessary.

When I got back in the house I knew I was in trouble. Walking on uneven surfaces has always put me into a tailspin and this was a doozy. My lower back started to ache and pinch and complain. It started disturbing my sleep. Two days later, the left leg was giving out on me. The problem kept grumbling away for two weeks despite everything I could throw at it — ice, heat, rest, exercise, coffee enemas, extra magnesium. Miriam was so happy about my other break-throughs that she didn't at first pay much attention to this new/old problem.

Finally, I made a stand. "I can't walk properly. I've done everything I can but I still can't walk straight."

"Oh," she said. "Well, let's see you walk." And I paraded up and down a few times.

"Hmm," she said. "There's something, but what? I want to measure." She measured each leg. "That's a surprise!" she said. "I'd never have guessed. Your right leg seems to be a whole inch shorter than your left. Up to half an inch isn't usually a problem, but a whole inch could throw out your gait quite a bit. In fact," she went on, "your sacrilization may even have developed as a result of this. Go and have a quarter of an

inch put on your shoe and see how that goes. We don't want to do too much at once."

So I did go and have my shoe adjusted. Cautiously I wore it around the house for a couple of hours. The next day I wore it for my walk. The next day I wore it all day. Without the shoe I could feel how the right side dragged down the left and how I rolled a bit as I walked. How many more surprises has my body got in store for me?

After fifty-one years, I know why running races was not my forte. And why I always walked so slowly no matter how I tried to hurry. When we see children struggling along in some way, why do we not look for physical reasons first? We are much too stuck on the power of the mind to affect physical performance and not stuck enough on the power of physical function to affect the mind.

Hormones

Just when you think you've taken the bull by the horns, something else happens. In my case, my estrogen flat-lined. Every hour on the hour, like Old Faithful, my body turned into a raging inferno. Nights became sweat-soaked sleeplessness. It's hard to describe the feeling that I was somehow being consumed into little gray ashes and black twisted cinders.

Fortunately, Dr. M had just swirled the cape in front of this bull herself as she sought to adjust her estrogen levels during menopause. In her opinion (and that of Dr. Alan Gaby in his book, *Preventing and Reversing Osteoporosis*), the best strategy would be to eat lots of soy products and use herbs to manage. Didn't work for her. Didn't work for me either. After another month of of little sleep, I was a frazzled rag.

Plan B for her and for me was to be a new estrogen prepa-ration called Tri-est, which contained percentages of estriol, etradial, and estrone similar to those naturally occurring in the body — that is, 80 percent, 10 percent, and 10 percent, respec-tively. Estriol is a weaker form of estrogen, but actually protects against cancer rather than promoting it, according to the stud-ies cited by Dr. Gaby. Naturally this preparation was *not* includ-ed under my drug plan. I took it and for a little while experi-enced a blessed sleep and much less sweating. Unfortunately, I also began to feel more and more lethargic and depressed.

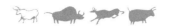

08/97 Chris had planted a squash vine on the compost heap out behind the deck fence. The vine had grown profusely. I had trained it with my bare hands to grow up the trellis. And yes, it does have something to do with menopause. A couple of weeks later, I went out to the deck for a breath of air after dinner and I leaned over the fence to examine the developing squash. My left elbow happened to lean on a prickly squash leaf. It hurt a bit. I moved off it and thought no more. My elbow developed a dark red swelling. It looked as if I had dipped my elbow in acid — and it felt that way too. The swelling spread. My family physician had never seen anything quite like it. Neither had anyone else. A cortisone cream failed to help. Then the swelling began to spread up my arm.

I took some peelings out to the compost heap and accidentally touched a finger to the squash vine. My finger immediately developed a swollen red rash. The next morning it had spread to the other fingers, and I was feeling quite ill as well as frightened. My appointment with Dr. M was on Monday, but I was afraid to wait over weekend, so I called her office and explained. They consulted with her and called back right away.

"Go back on the licorice!' she advised. I had tried the licorice treatment, per Dr. D'Adamo, a couple of months before. It consisted of a solid licorice extract (a black tar-like substance) accompanied by potassium and methionine. A quarter of a teaspoon in water, 300-400 mg potassium and 500 mg of methionine at 10:00 a.m. and 3:00 p.m. After only a couple of days, it had made quite a difference to the pain and brain fog. It helped me cope with chemicals much better. I had used it for three months, run out of supplies, and decided to give it a rest before I became allergic to the stuff.

I had no licorice, nor was any available at local stores, but a friend who had tried the licorice treatment, though it had made her diarrhea worse, not only had some but she also

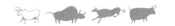

had the methionine to go with it. I had some potassium. I was in business. I mixed up a dose, and within an hour the swelling was visibly less. It was amazing! But this started me thinking. Since the licorice helps the liver clear chemicals, what was overloading my liver? I had been reading Dr. Gaby's book and learned that oral estrogen had to be converted in the liver to a form that the body could use. Perhaps that was it — my liver couldn't metabolize the estrogen.

By the time I got to Dr. M, having taken the licorice every day, my rash was fading but by no means gone. Dr. M concurred that it was the oral estrogen and prescribed an estrogen patch. The transdermal form does not need to be converted in the liver. My body heaved a sigh of relief when I slapped on the patch, but it still didn't feel great. The patch is not Tri-est.

I had a friend with the same problem metabolizing the oral estrogen, and she wanted the Tri-est instead of the usual patch. She phoned the pharmacy where the oral Tri-est was compounded. Yes, they could make a cream form. Off we went to our family doctor for the prescription. Then off to the fax machine to send it.

When the cream arrived a couple of days later, I slathered on the required 1/4 tsp. My body felt even more relief. This felt much, much better, more normal. Meanwhile, my elbow and arm were rapidly healing, though the ugly red marks took several months to fade to brown and then disappear. The scary addendum to this is that another woman on oral estrogen had a much more frightening episode when we were going through this. She went blind from swelling, which impinged on the optic nerve, and ended up in intensive care. Fortunately, the problem was figured out in time so that she recovered her health and sight.

I started to sleep better and sweat less. The next step was to add progesterone in the 3 percent cream form. The usual method was to use it for a week or so a month. I tried that,

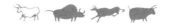

felt better for the week, and then felt really rotten discontinuing it. My friend was using it every day. Dr M. approved the strategy, so I started slathering on two creams twice day.

A quarter of a teaspoon doesn't seem like much until you try spreading it on yourself. Remember that you must use approved areas of tender skin, but not breast, and you must rotate the areas used.

It took a few notes stuck on the bathroom mirror until I got a system organized that I could remember easily. I also had one cream formulation changed so that I only needed 1/8 of a teaspoon. That helped too. Talk about slipping through the day!

I thought things might level out then, but no, my legs started cramping severely in the night. The long bones would ache fiercely. Sleep was out of the question. Of course, I resorted to my old friend, magnesium, but that backfired and made the pain worse. What was going on?

According to Dr. Gaby (whose book by the way helped me solve my puffy gums using 1 mg extra per day of folic acid, thus surprising my dental hygienist and dentist all to pieces), progesterone is necessary for rebuilding bone cells. Hmmmm. Rebuilding bone. Bone needs calcium. Calcium deficiency causes ... pain in the long bones and leg cramps. This brainwave, one painful 3:00 a.m., caused me to get up and take an extra calcium. Within half an hour I was asleep.

It took awhile to regulate the calcium magnesium balance so that I could make it through the whole night. There were a few calcium/magnesium IVs instead of magnesium alone. I finally began taking a more normal balance (1:1) of calcium and magnesium, although with chemical exposure and such, the need for extra magnesium would reassert itself. The balancing act became more routine.

Eating Right for Your Type

Why rest on my laurels? The main problem was still not resolved. I was still disabled. The pain still fluctuated unpredictably. Dr. M recommended another test and another book. Jeffrey Bland's book, *The 20 Day Rejuvenation Diet Program*, pulls together a great deal of the new paradigm in a systematic way. I ignored the diet. I already had as much as I could stomach that way, literally. I did the questionnaire and headed into the chapters indicated by my scores. "Pain and Inflammation" seemed like a good place to start.

The first thing that leaped out at me was "calcium band-aids." According to the book, everywhere there is pain and inflammation, the body lays down "calcium bandaids." This seemed to fit with what was happening in my physical therapy. These deposits were being released, and my detoxification strategies, to say nothing of extra magnesium, were required to flush them out of my system. And since I had had inflammation practically everywhere, there were — no had been — innumerable "calcium bandaids" to unstick.

I discovered that I was already following almost all of Bland's recommendations for pain and inflammation, but that wasn't the part Dr. M had in mind. The chapter on "Toxins from Within" and "Detoxifying" were more what she was interested in. In these, Bland describes some tests — the

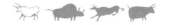

Comprehensive Digestive and Stool Analysis (CDSA), the Intestinal Permeability Test, and the Liver Detoxification Panel. Dr. M would like me, ideally, to have them all. My VISA account disagreed. The CDSA alone would cost almost $400. I was starting to run out of resources, but then again, what price health? After hemming and hawing and scrimping, rereading Bland and putting up with the pain, I finally gave in. Hurry up and wait. It would take three weeks to get results.

10/97 In the meantime (my theme song), I had another book to read, a book by the son of a doctor who pioneered the licorice treatment, Dr. D'Adamo. Since the licorice came close to saving my bacon, reading the book was the least I could do. His *Eat Right for Your Type* became my companion. Dr. D'Adamo's theory is that the more primitive your blood type, the more primitive your diet should be. It is based on some scientific evidence that certain foods cause unhealthy changes in certain blood types. Blood types range from O, which is the most ancient, through A and B to AB which is the most recent. I'm an O. D'Adamo thinks that people with that type get into trouble when they eat more modern foods like grains and dairy products. Roots 'r' us. Meat, too. Dr. M recommended I try it. She was doing so herself.

So, out of my poor old rotary diet went a few more foods — rye and wheat, barley and oats. However, I kept in the spelt/kamut bread as Dr. D'Adamo and others like Dr. Ali figured that these were different enough and ancient enough to be tolerated. I adjusted to the losses with more roots — yucca, eddoes, and jerusalem artichokes (my sister just had in a bumper organic crop). I managed to survive but my weight was a little precarious.

When the CDSA results came in, it showed that I was not digesting my food due to a lack of stomach acid. I was also low in lactobacillus. And I had an overgrowth of Candida parapsilosas.

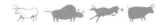

So ... more betaine de hydochloride with pepsin before meals and pancreatin half an hour after. Chew really, really, reeeally well! Increase lactobacillus powder (acidophillus) and get the kind with fructooligasaccarides (FOS) which feeds the friendly bacteria, not the unfriendly. Increasing stomach acid would also make the gut more acidic and, therefore, less hospitable to candida. The acidophillus would help crowd it out, too.

The third item recommended by the test was uva ursi, identified as a specific against this particular type of candida. Dr. M was at a loss about this herb, so she suggested I find someone knowledgeable about it. I trotted off to a local nutrition shop where there was someone trained to use a gizmo called a Biotron which uses electrical resistance at acupuncture points to determine whether an item is beneficial for you or not. The first order of business was to take a baseline reading. Then we gathered up all the uva ursi preparations and tested them one by one until we found one that produced the most favorable reading. While I was there, I had tested a few other things D'Adamo lists for healing the gut. Aloe vera was negative. So was astalagus and alfalfa. So was wheat. Potatoes, to my sceptical delight, came up positive.

On to the uva ursi with caution because it is causes water retention and is hard on the kidneys. I made sure to include ginger, cranberries, and a little extra potassium in my rotation.

Garlic was also highlighted by the CDSA as a useful specific, so after a month on the uva ursi, I went back, tested it out and threw that in too.

Whether because of diet or gut treatment or both, my physical abilities started to improve. Before, I would try to clean the bathroom or dust another room and I would be flattened for a week. My son had been doing all the housework. Now I could do two rooms a week or in a really good week, three. Sometimes, of course, I still couldn't do any. The high points were getting higher and the lows not so low.

Celiac Disease

The ice storm of the century hit eastern Ontario, and I was terrified, not just by the storm, which was scary enough as the trees around us came down all night like dump truck loads of ice-covered spears. Trees cracked like bombs going off. The devastation visible next morning was frightening. More than all that, I was afraid of having to go to a shelter. I could barely cope in my own sheltered environment with my own quiet bed and my own specialized food and the facilities to do all my detoxification treatments. If I had to go to a shelter in a school gymnasium or something, it would be extremely hard on me. I sympathized with the seniors reported resisting going to shelters despite very cold conditions in their homes. The gods smiled on me. The power went out for four hours ... and came back on, went out for another four hours . . . and came back on. That was it. Some terror over the basement flooding and a trip out to borrow a generator but that was it. We didn't even have to resort to using the fireplace, which would have given me problems.

01/98 My older son was not so lucky. His power was out for fifteen days, so he and his cat, Lochland, came to camp with us. Our cat did not approve and tended to pee whenever she caught sight of Lochland so we set up a changing of the

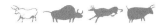

guard. One cat under room arrest while the other had the freedom of the house and yard (once the hanging limbs were no longer a danger.) The only problem was that Lochland is a hefty cat, unlike our tiny one. In order to change the guard, someone had to corral Lochland and put him in Mike's room. When Mike went back north to help with the ice storm effort, I threw out my back and Lochland had to board at the vet for a few days. Poor puss. Poor me. Mike's power was restored but then it was discovered his deep well pump was split and so another week went by as he camped in his place and wrangled water in jugs.

When things calmed down, the 'flu hit. I guess the stress made everyone more vulnerable, and Chris brought home a doozy of a case from work. I made chicken soup, and somehow the spoons got mixed up. I got one he had licked, thereby inoculating myself with the plague. The flu turned the bull into 'superbull' and me into a trampled mess.

Two weeks later, another kind of 'bug' hit. Canada Pension Disability sent me for a Functional Ability Evaluation (FAE). This is the new way that compensation plans have of harassing their dependents. For half an hour, I had to review my whole case again for the benefit of a physiotherapist and a kinesiologist. Then I was scheduled for three and a half hours of bending, lifting, reaching, pushing, pulling, gripping, squatting, and walking on a treadmill. Because of the arrhythmias, I was hooked up to a halter monitor. With every test, the pain reaction came quicker and harder. I lasted less than a minute on the treadmill. We took a number of breaks for me to lie down, and we stopped for lunch, even though it was an hour early. They decided to send me home.

I planned for a magnesium IV that afternoon to try to minimize the damage. I got home and took a salt and soda bath. By bedtime, I was ready for the hot and cold packs. A bad night, up and down for heat and ice. When I woke, I immediately realized I shouldn't have. Eyeballs too sore to

Celiac Disease

move, pain down sides and front of neck making it hard to move, knife-like pains around ribs making it hard to breathe, arrhythmias, pain like hot wires down both arms, hands like stiff, painful baseball gloves, pain from chin to pelvis making it painful to stand, sciatica down right leg making walking painful. I was a mess. I spent the day on ice and heat packs, propped in the least painful position. I took magnesium and vitamin C. I called the clinic to tell them the shape I was in. If had had a 'teleporter' from Star Trek, I would have sent myself to the office of the bureaucrat in charge of my case. I did try to phone and see if they had any way of providing some treatment for my situation. I had to content myself with drafting a letter in my head to my elected government representative. There was nothing to do but suffer.

Four days later, I heard the fuel oil truck filling the furnace oil tank. I usually smell a few fumes from the truck and so didn't think too much until I went to the top of the stairs for something and smelled a strong stink of oil. I went down a few steps toward the basement and felt panic. The basement smelled strongly of fuel oil. The seal on the oil gauge had crumbled, allowing a couple quarts of oil to spill over the side of the tank. Through the increasing haze of an allergic reaction, I called the company who promised to send someone.

My recollection of the next 24 hours is rather patchy. I remember arriving at a friend's house with my nightgown and toothbrush in a tote bag. I don't really remember driving myself there. I remember the bad night worrying about Chris and Matt home with the poisonous stink and the windows wide to the early March rawness. I remember going home in the morning to have another allergic reaction despite the oil having been cleaned up. The stuff they used to clean up smelled almost as bad as the oil. I called for another clean-up.

At physical therapy, she said I looked like a deer caught

in the headlights. My doctor agreed as he administered a magnesium IV. The next trip home was no better. I called for the furnace company once again. By this time they considered me a real pain in the butt. I sat in the car sick as a dog while they did their best. Then, too exhausted to care anymore, I managed a dash to our bedroom, which was furthest from the spill. I spent the next 24 hours curled in a ball, practically unmoving. As I write this, my body is registering the experience over again. I don't want to stress myself any more. Suffice it to say, for the next six weeks, I did every detox procedure in the book including extra glutathione, salt and soda baths, the licorice treatment, coffee enemas, extra vitamin C.

Of course, bad luck runs in packs, not just threes. The next week, my car, which my older son had been using, blew its headgasket and cracked its engine block. We took him back his own 15-year-old vehicle fondly named Myrtle for her green color (which I had been driving and on whom I had just spent $150 to have the remains of a mouse removed from her heater.) Two days later, in a later snowstorm on his way home over a road unplowed because of funding cuts, Myrtle did a doughnut and took out her front headlight and grill on a guardrail which rendered her too expensive to repair.

On our return the day we took Myrtle back to Mike, we came home to a flooding basement because one sump pump had broken down. Oh goody, stink *and* mold. Two days after that, on the other end of the oil tank, a small gasket gave out and we had a second spill much smaller than the first, a cup or so. Then we discovered that the carport pillars were rotten at the bottom and the roof was in danger!

I'm beginning to laugh because it all seems so impossibly bizarre. When I told a friend about our tribulations, she thought I was pulling her leg. The Fates were yanking hard on ours! When I told Dr. M about it all, she ordered up a multi-nutrient IV, which helped me recover a bit more easily.

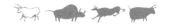

You think that's it? Wrong. At the end of May, we had construction done to install the connection to the new municipal water line. Unfortunately, the construction messed up our sump outlet, and we had another flood in a violent thunderstorm, one of many that characterized this season. The dampness stirred up the oil fumes again, so Chris tore out more wall, removed flooring, and we rented an ozone generator which ran in the basement for a week and made a significant difference. Then the lawn tractor died. My husband's blood sugar levels went seriously out of whack. Stress or the fuel oil exposure or both?

My CDSA test had shown that I handle stress well. Darn good thing! Oh, and I managed to go to Sudbury schools for a week to read poems from my new book-in-progress for children, *How Do You Wrestle a Goldfish?* That was a psychological boost, even if it was rather poor timing physically. A couple of other workshops with Pat, along with a lecture and presentations at Indigo Books, made me feel I had a life, even if it was a struggle.

A good omen appeared. Because another patient had found a normalization of leg length during an insurance-mandated physical, my physical therapist remeasured my legs and found that I too had gone from a one-inch discrepancy, a year ago, to a normal 1/4 inch now. The shoemaker was amazed when I returned to ask him to remove the lifts he had installed on all my right shoes. He commented that this never happened. How had it happened? I explained, as she had to me, that the discrepancy must have been myofascial in origin rather than skeletal. The myofascial work had put it right.

07/98 I had come to expect that any chemical exposure would cause my gut to shut down for at least ten days and maybe up to three weeks with big exposures. During the summer with windows wide open, no events to attend, there

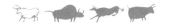

seemed much less reason for any reaction. For part of July, I felt really miserable, even though my range of motion had improved and I was struggling to extend what I could do around the house. I felt 'down in the dumps,' not interested in much. My gut would not work more than one week a month. I was very happy not to be in the kind of pain I had had. All this sounds very contradictory and confusing. That's how it felt, too. My friends in the reading group were in similar situations. Sometimes a little better, sometimes worse.

When I felt miserable over Chris' holiday, even my physical therapist made an oblique comment about psychology. Chris and I disagree over what is a holiday. His idea is to become a hermit for two weeks and paint. My idea is to become social and cook for friends and visit. It's only natural since he goes out to work every day and I stay home. I thought I had solved it by having various friends for lunch the week before his holiday so that I wouldn't feel deprived when we became hermits. He compromised, and we went one day up to Michael's to help him with a repair job. Of course, that turned out to be the hottest day of the year with the worst air pollution index. I ended up driving around in the smog to stinky lumber yards and hardware stores to pick up bits that became necessary as the job progressed. I had to agree with Chris that staying home seemed terribly attractive.

Then Chris' holidays were over and I still felt miserable. My friends and I began to run down the list of things we had done for something we had missed. Dr. Sherry Rogers says that 90 per cent of the patients get well using 20 percent of the armamentarium. Here I was, having done 90 percent of the strategies, and I was a long way from well yet.

To date I had implemented the following strategies:

1. a rotation diet of mostly organic foods with known aller gens excluded
2. a diet with no sugar, caffeine, alcohol, or additives

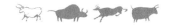

3. a diet carefully balanced for fat/protein/carbohydrate
4. a supplementation of the diet with a balanced program of vitamins, minerals, essential fatty acids, and fiber
5. aids to digestion such as betaine de hydrochloride with pepsin and pancreatin
6. a supplementation of the hormones DHEA, estrogen, and progesterone to normal levels
7. a clean environment at home (well, most of the time)
8. an avoidance of chemical exposures as much as possible
9. detoxification strategies
10. treatments for parasites and yeast
11. relaxation strategies
12. exercise regimen
13. physical therapy

Phew!!! What more could a person do?

Despite all this, I had severe constipation most of the time; a rash on my elbow, face, thigh, buttock, and hairline; nutrient deficiencies; weight loss; muscle pain, spasm, wasting and weakness; neurological symptoms such as tingling, twitching, crawling sensations, pain, and sometimes headache; sleep disturbance; fatigue; food and chemical sensitivities; hypoglycemic episodes; arrhthmias at times; back jam-ups; occasional confusion and brain fog; restlessness; and — surprise — anxiety and depressed mood.

I began to worry that perhaps I had a cancer, so I began taking a protein supplement suggested by Dr. M, Immunocal. A friend's mother with leukemia had been taking it with some good results. The protein supplement seemed to give me a bit more energy and hypoglycemic episodes became less.

Then came the muffin. Chris brought home a whole wheat muffin from the bakery which made the spelt/kamut bread I was using on one day of my rotation. The muffin had no nuts or raisins, a little carob and a little maple syrup. Nothing too allergenic, but I didn't want to eat it. I did want

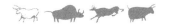

to eat it. It sat on the counter calling to me. After a couple of hours, I gave in and ate it.

That was either a big mistake or a big step forward, depending how you look at it. That night, it felt like a big mistake — cramps, bloating, pain, severe pain. My gut which had been working fine for two weeks went into conniptions. And when the enemas worked, I was reminded of something I had read about celiac disease.

One of my friends had been on about gluten sensitivity. We'd all tried giving it up at various stages. Some books said spelt/kamut was enough different to be okay. Others said no way. My allergy test had come back with wheat okay, just the mold that could grow on it might be a problem. The Biotron testing had indicated that wheat was not good for me, but, oddly, the spelt/kamut tested neutral. The descriptions I'd read of celiac disease always emphasized diarrhea, so we had already decided that wasn't it. Besides our diets were so restricted already. I didn't know what to think.

By chance — or serendipity — I had visited my aunt and uncle to pick out a 'chainsaw' sculpture for Matthew's birthday. At that time, my aunt mentioned that her daughter, my first cousin, had a lot of allergies. "She eats mainly chicken and rice," said my aunt. Hmmm. I asked for my cousin's address, intending to share information. When I called back to see if the sculpture was ready, my aunt mentioned that her daughter's problem was really gluten. Gluten!! Barley, rye, oats, and wheat!

If you encounter something three times, pay attention! It took my gut ten days to start functioning properly again. By then, I was becoming more certain. Then began the usual panic of sustaining life while learning a new diet. The spelt/kamut bread was the caloric mainstay of one day of my rotation. What was I going to substitute?

I called my local health food store which I knew carried a full line of gluten-free products. It just so happened that the

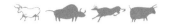

president of the local Celiac Support Group was in the store. We arranged to meet. She gave me some pamphlets, etc. and recommended a website.

When I woke in the middle of that night, I went to the Internet found www.celiac.com. The articles there confirmed that celiac symptoms can take many guises and be associated with many diseases, including rheumatoid arthritis and chronic fatigue! It referred to an article in *The Lancet* (February 1996) which dealt with neurological symptoms like muscle weakness, muscle wasting, poor coordination, and balance. Maybe I was getting somewhere! The website also had lists of safe foods and additives as well as foods and additives to avoid. There was a caution on soy milk! Barley enzymes! There went the protein and calories in another breakfast! Baking soda could also be contaminated. I couldn't even brush my teeth safely. (It makes my head ache a bit just writing all this down.) I downloaded the information for my friends in the reading group.

We had a gluten-free lunch (lamb borscht) and discussed what to do. The information on testing said that neither the small intestine biopsy nor the blood screening was very conclusive. Besides, one had to continue to eat gluten until the tests. I knew that an invasive test like the biopsy would be very hard on me. I didn't know where to have the blood screening done. I wasn't willing to eat gluten for any longer if it meant my gut wouldn't work, especially when I read that the main risk for undiagnosed, middle-aged celiacs was lymphoma of the small intestine! I might as well just hold down the exclamation key for this whole section!!!!!!!!!!!

Celiac disease means that you do not have the enzyme to digest gluten. That causes damage to the villi in the intestine which causes lactose intolerance, which causes leaky gut, which causes nutrient deficiencies and more allergies, so you end up with poor liver function and immune complexes parked in inappropriate places all over your body — and

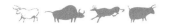

that's literally a big pain. Talk about a cascade of symptoms!

I'm going for the blood screening in a day or so. I'm trying to construct a gluten-free diet that will sustain me. I'm keeping on with all my strategies because with the possible damage to repair, my body is going to need all the help it can get over the next year. Becoming healthy is a life-long pursuit, I have learned. In another year, I hope, I'll have a party! I may have several.

Afterword

Early one morning, up writing some of the last bits of this book, I took a break and picked up a magazine which had a review of Rosemary Sullivan's biography of Margaret Atwood, accompanied by an interview with the biographer. In the interview, Rosemary regrets her childless state and consoles herself with Margaret Atwood's pronouncement that there are three aspects to her life — job, family, and writing — and that a woman can only manage any two of them successfully. That was like a floodlight illuminating the dimensions and components of the huge bull I had been lifting, the myths and premises that had frustrated me for so long. They range from the personal and idiosyncratic through literary, economic, gender, medical, environmental, psychological, and spiritual. I've probably missed some.

The medical myths are the most obvious. Allopathic surgical and pharmaceutical medicine is great in a crisis of injury or attack by microorganisms. It can keep you alive to fight another day, but its emphasis on the critical care mode of squashing symptoms makes it ill-suited for long-term problems. Naturopathic or environmental medicine might not be able to offer instant solutions, but it is developing wonderful strategies for listening to the body's symptoms as it responds to its supply of air, water, food, and toxic add-ons. The ideal would be to have both allopathic and orthomolecular medicine available and

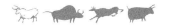

working together in complementary fashion. The possibilities are exciting.

The economic myths are pretty obvious as well. It is an often-quoted statistic in the disability compensation systems that people who do not return to work within a year have a very low probability of doing so. This is translated into a drive to get people back to work as quickly as possible, no matter what the means. In the light of my experience, it might be better to look differently at those people who do not heal in the usual time for the given injury. Perhaps we should wonder why they are still ill and perhaps look for physical reasons for the problem? Maybe they are not back to work because they are still too sick. The desire of people to work and be productive is seriously and grossly under-rated.

Gender myths follow closely on the heels of the medical and economic. Because many medical trials and investigations involve only men, the understanding gathered may not reflect women's realities. Because economic systems follow the patterns of men's lives more closely, women are blamed for not fitting the models. Again we should be asking where the models are falling down for women and what can be done to change the models not how women can be physically altered to accommodate the models. In fact, the models are not kind to men either and changes could benefit everyone.

Psychology has become a dumping ground for things we do not understand. Psychology has become a place to make up intellectual theories to explain the effects of physical problems. There is a place for psychology and it is in examining the strategies people use in solving problems and in relating to one another. It is in teaching people to use these strategies, thereby becoming more independent and successful.

Spirituality has been warped similarly by the human tendency to idolize or demonize what is feared or not understood. Spirituality, instead, can recognize that we do not understand everything in the universe. It is much vaster

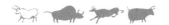

than we are. Spirituality can help us recognize that fear is a survival mechanism for making us cautious around what we do not understand. Spirituality has been warped into systems for excluding others from the 'chosen,' instead of systems for helping people find balance, wonder, enrichment and harmony.

I'm not too sure about the literary myths. I survived the ones from the fifties that declared that women probably couldn't write or otherwise be creative because they didn't have penises. Then there were the creative-type-as-mad-person myths. Then there were the artistic snobbisms which apportioned status to art depending on its genre. After that came such things as creative success measured in terms of fame or money. There was the denigration of teaching. These are just a few. None of them are helpful. Indeed they are destructive to many. Science and creativity depend a great deal more than they would like to admit on trial and error and serendipity. Trying and learning are the great things — the joyous, positive things.

All of these systems have led to unjustified negative judgements being made about all sorts of people. I have felt the power of these labels — daughter of a suicide, hypochondriac, nervous wreck, overachieving woman, working mother, poor person, bankrupt, malingerer, shirker, drain on the system, hysteric, obsessive, neurotic, Type A, workaholic, malcontent, unbeliever, fraud, menopausal woman, layabout, only a children's writer, only a poet, etc., etc.

These myths are the bull. I have tried to lift them, temporarily been squashed, then stood up proud to have overcome the weight of pain and guilt. I have been ill probably more or less all my life, and yet I have worked, raised a family, and written, as well as I could. One tiny little part of me may mourn what might have been, but most of me celebrates arriving at this moment.

Reading List

I wish for your sake there was only one book to read to help yourself achieve better health. I read many but found no such one. Here I have listed the best books I consulted on back pain, fibromyalgia, environmental illness, and general well-being. These are not the only books available, not by a long shot. There are plenty. If you want to read more, consult my guide through the maze of health literature, *Reading To Heal*, which reviews over 50 titles. However, you may not want to plow through any more than necessary. The following books I do consider to be necessary, though each book in this bibliography has its strengths and weaknesses. Each author looks at the problem from a different perspective. This is both their value and limitation.

Value because each person with these problems has a different history, a different body, and so requires a different specific treatment. You may find clues, parts of the problem, parts of the solution, in each book.

Limitation because any one of these books may leave you with enthusiasm but not all of the strategies you need to solve your own particular problems. It is a complex task to sort out what is happening in your body, so don't be discouraged if one book does not do it all.

It may appear that I have neglected books on psychology in this bibliography. I am safely assuming that anyone reading my book has already had psychology stuffed in by the buck-etful, though every book in the list has some psychology in it. Any psychology book I could recommend would have to be called "Flying in the Face of Received Wisdom and Not Melting Your Wings Off." I can't seem to find it listed anywhere.

For convenience, I've divided the books into two categories, basic books on nutritional healing and specific books on fibromyalgia. The books on nutrition supercede the syndrome-specific discussions which tend to repeat the same information and hold out dubious promises of recovery. And I've followed the list with the plan I have used for establishing "Reading To Heal" book clubs and self-help groups in my community. I encourage you to do the same in yours. Helping friends to heal themselves is, in my experience, healthy.

Books on Nutritional Healing

Ali, Dr. Majid. *The Canary and Chronic Fatigue*. Bloomfield, NJ: The Institute of Preventive Medicine, 1995.

This book is essential for anyone suffering the effects of chemical overload. Chapter Seven on the origin of the problems and the chapters on nutrient protocols are most interesting and helpful. It may be worthwhile to show these to your physician.

Balch, James F., M.D. and Phyllis A., C.N.C. *Prescription for Nutritional Healing*. Garden City, NJ: Avery Publishing Group Inc., 1997.

This book has a great deal of interesting information on nutritional strategies, though they tend to be amazingly similar for widely varying conditions. Still, it can help you with figuring out the rotary diet and your allergies. *Prescription for Dietary Wellness*, also written by James and

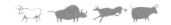

Phyllis Balch, has a good list of herbs and their effects on systems in the body.

Bland, Jeffrey. *The 20-day Rejuvenation Diet Program*. New Canaan, CT: Keats Publishing, 1997.

A good overview of nutritional healing with clear explanations of the problems and sensible discussions of nutritional treatments.

Crook, William, M.D. *The Yeast Connection*. Jackson, TN: Professional Books Inc., 1989.

For those suspecting a Candida problem, this is an important book.

Hoffer, Abram, M.D. *Hoffer's Laws of Natural Nutrition: Eating Well for Pure Health*. Kingston, ON: Quarry Health Books, 1995.

For anyone who wants to start on a nutrient supplementation program, this book sets out a process for discovering what suits you best. It's easier said than done, but, if you persist, Hoffer's process should work.

Rapp, Doris, M.D. *Is This Your Child?* New York, NY: Random House, 1991.

This book offers well-researched information on the causes, effects, and treatments of allergies, with excellent descriptions of diets that help you sort out the problem more quickly. Traditional allergists may disagree but patients obviously have their own opinions.

Rajhathy, Judit. *Free To Fly*. Halifax, NS: New World Publishing, 1995.

This book is a fictionalized account of going through the nutritional process. Because the protagonist's problems are so easily and quickly resolved, for those of us whose problems persist, this book can become discouraging.

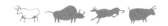

Rogers, Dr. Sherry. *Wellness Against All Odds.* Syracuse, NY: Prestige Publishing, 1994.

For anyone with allergies, chemical sensitivities, pain from bad backs or other areas, this book is quite enlightening as well as hopeful. Dr. Rogers explains a great deal about minerals, especially magnesium, and their functions in the body. Another of her books, Tired or Toxic, goes into more technical detail for doctors, but has a useful discussion of detoxification processes which may help speed recovery.

Sears, Barry. *The Zone.* New York, NY: Harper Collins, 1996.

The author, a biochemist, explains a diet he developed to deal with his own family history of heart disease. His diet intends to balance all the elements of diet to provoke the body's proper hormonal response to food, a regimen tested and found successful by people with heart disease, diabetes, rheumatoid arthritis and many other conditions, as well as by Olympic competitors.

Weil, Andrew, M.D. *Spontaneous Healing.* New York: Alfred A. Knopf, 1995.

The author describes a variety of alternative methods which have helped many people, but he warns against the side-effects of some. The book has considerable information on herbs, vitamins and minerals, but I was especially interested in Chapter 2 on osteopathy, which deals with the spinal and myofascial problems we accumulate over time and as a result of injuries.

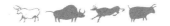

Clinical Books about Fibromyalgia

Chaitow, Leon. *Muscle Pain: What Causes It, How It Feels and What To Do About It.* New York, NY: Harper, 1996.
   The author explains the usual treatments that may help to relieve symptoms somewhat but are not a long-term cure.

Conley, Edward. *America Exhausted: Breakthrough Treatments of Fatigue and Fibromyalgia.* Flint, MI: Vitality Press, 1997.
   He does address diet and digestion.

Ediger, Beth. *Coping with Fibromyalgia (Fibrositis).* Toronto: LRH Publications, 1991.
   This early booklet covers diagnosis, symptoms, then-current treatments, and coping skills.

Goldberg, Burton and the editors of Alternative Medicine Digest. *Chronic Fatigue, Fibromyalgia & Environmental Illness.* Tiburton, CA: Future Medicine Publishing, 1998.
   This book contains many case histories and tantalizing hints about alternative treatments, but just as you start to feel excited about a treatment, the section ends and you find many products named that are exclusive to the practitioners so that there is a feeling of an 'infomercial' about it all.

Goldengerg, Don L., M.D. *Chronic Illness & Uncertainty: A Personal & Professional Guide to Poorly Understood Syndromes, What We Do Know and Don't Know about Fibromyalgia.* Newton Lower Falls, MA: Dorset, 1996.
   In a diary form, the author revisits in psychological and pharmaceutical treatments.

Goldstein, Jay A. *Betrayal by the Brain: The Neurologic Basis of Chronic Fatigue Syndrome, Fibromyalgia Syndrome and Related Neural Network Disorders.* New York, NY: Haworth Press, 1996.
   The approach is very technical and oriented to pharmaceutical treatments.

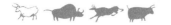

Lorig, K.; Fries, J.F. *The Arthritis Helpbook: A Tested Self-management Program for Coping with Arthritis and Fibromyalgia*. Reading, MA: Addison-Wesley, 1995.

The usual advice on exercise and pain management.

MacIlwain, Harris, M.D, and Bruce, Debra. *Fibromyalgia Handbook*. New York, NY: Henry Holt, 1996.

In reviewing this book, I am reminded by the contents that a large part of the energy of anyone ill with these problems must go to dealing with compensation battles, the strain on interpersonal relationships and the attack on self-image. Dealing with your health is almost regarded as a minor consideration.

Morgan, Sarah L. *The Essential Arthritis Cookbook: Kitchen Basics for People with Arthritis, Fibromyalgia and Other Chronic Pain and Fatigue*. Mankato, MN: Appletree, 1995.

The advice given here by traditional dietitians did not help me.

Russell, I.J. *Clinical Overview and Pathogenesis of the Fibromyalgia Syndrome, Myofascial Pain Syndrome and Other Pain Syndromes*. New York, NY: Haworth Press, 1996.

Bio-individuality makes it almost impossible to deliver what this book attempts, a universal explanation.

Starlanyl, Devin J., M.D. *The Fibromyalgia Advocate*. Oakland, CA: New Harbinger, 1998.
Starlanyl, Devin J., M.D. and Copeland, Mary Ellen. *Fibromyalgia & Chronic Myofascial Pain Syndrome.*. Oakland, CA: New Harbinger, 1996.

These two books contain useful information on the FM Impact Assessment, for example, and a wide description of possible symptoms as well as brief descriptions of some treatment modalities. Since Starlanyl herself has the problem, there are some personal comments.

Teitelbaum, J. *From Fatigued to Fantastic.* Garden City, NJ: Avery Publishing, 1996.

> This book almost made the "A list" because it contains lots of valuable information on the nutritional approach.

Williamson, Miyam Ehrlich. *Fibromyalgia: A Comprehensive Approach.* New York, NY: Walker & Company, 1996.

Williamson, Miyam Ehrlich. *The Fibromyalgia Relief Book: 213 Ideas for Improving Your Quality of Life.* New York, NY: Walker and Co., 1996.

> The first book by Williamson tries to cover all the bases in a simplified way and includes 10 case histories with lots of hints but little depth, the usual problem with the 'comprehensive' approach. His ideas for improving 'quality of life' may be useful.

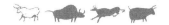

Reading to Heal:
Setting Up a Health Book Reading Group

Today there is a wealth of information available about medical conditions and medical strategies — so much that our family doctors can only keep up to certain parts. People with problems can — and often must — become quite expert on their own conditions by reading as much as possible.

However, I remember how useful it was to have a buddy with whom to discuss the books. Why not a reading group just for books on health? To help out, I had *Hoffer's Laws of Natural Nutrition*, a bibliography of other helpful books, twenty-five years teaching experience, and five years with a pleasure-reading group. Health care professionals in my community, namely my physiotherapist and osteopath, passed along the names of their patients, and soon we had a reading group up and running.

Before the first meeting, I labored over a code of ethics. Judy and I realized that we could only offer our own experience and book references, not diagnose, urge treatment, or take responsibility for one another's decisions. We aren't doctors. We are reading buddies.

The other concern was power inequities. How would very ill people feel about reading with well people, or with professional caregivers, or with those with goods or services to sell? I decided to keep the group small, six to eight, and relatively homogeneous. I ended up with two groups and then three groups. It seems like an idea whose time has come.

Dr. Hoffer's book takes giant steps that can be filled in through other books on diet, allergies, toxicity, specific conditions, and so on. Although our reading-to-heal groups are just getting started, already members feel the difference. They are taking back some control and, as an added bonus, finding some answers. Just what we book addicts knew all along — the power of books.

Reading List

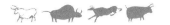

Reading To Heal Code of Ethics

We are trying to improve our own health through educating ourselves, not prying into the health of others.

No one in the group may presume to decide for anyone else. Each person must decide, perhaps in consultation with a nutritional health care professional, what is needed. We are not doctors or nutritional consultants.

We can offer our own experience.

We can offer references to other material.

We can offer interpretations of the books we read.

We cannot take responsibility for another's decisions or actions.

We must take responsibility for our own health, decisions and actions.

Helpful Hints for Starting and Running a Reading To Heal Group

1. Limit your numbers to about eight people.

2. Give members a month to read *Hoffer's Laws of Natural Nutrition.*

3. The meeting location should be as non-toxic as possible. Evaluate after the first meeting.

4. Take as many meetings per book as the group wants.

5. Don't be afraid to adjust the meetings to your groups needs — eliminate a hazardous weather month or a busy month for holidays, etc. Be comfortable with your schedule.

6. At each meeting, go around the circle and give each person a chance to comment on aspects of the book, such as: things especially noticed, helpful parts, difficult or confusing issues, personal experiences related to the book, or comparisons with other books.

Reading List

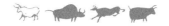

7. Take turns choosing the next book or come to a consensus.

8. This group is for the benefit of the members. Arrange it to suit your needs.

Reading To Heal Group Evaluation

MEETINGS: (Once a month or at group's discretion)

Appropriate: _____ frequency _____ location _____ length _____ time

Comments: _____

SIZE: (4-8)

How many in group? _____ _____ Appropriate _____ Too many _____ Too few

Comments: _____

BOOK CHOICES: (From bibliography)

__ helpful (e.g. _____)
__ not helpful (e.g._____)
__ too expensive (e.g. _____)

Comments: _____

DISCUSSION: (Round the group)

__ helpful   __ not helpful
__ too directed   __ not directed enough
__ open-minded   __ coercive

Comments: _____

EFFECTS:

__ tried some strategies   __ did not try any new strategies
__ felt more hopeful   __ felt discouraged
__ felt supported   __ felt left out
__ noticed positive/negative results of some strategies
__ generated more support in family/friends/caregivers
__ sought help of professional in nutritional/environmental therapy

Comments: _____

Reading List

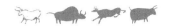

Remember always that in addition to considerable reading your recovery may take a long time, lots of energy, careful observation, patience, and persistence. If one strategy fails, it may need to be combined with another rather than discarded. Keep anything that helps even a little. Accumulate those helpful strategies until you experience good health once again.

Acknowledgements

Thanks first to my doctor of environmental medicine, here identified as Dr. M to prevent her from being overwhelmed with requests, who was the one who 'analyzed the bull' for me and encouraged me to take it by the horns, as she had herself. If she had not been brave and clever enough to stand up for what she believed in — the approach of clinical ecology or orthomolecular medicine or whatever you choose to call it — I might not be alive and writing this book. How can you thank someone for that? I can only acknowledge that this is the way it is.

Thanks to my family physician, who has always been supportive, willing to implement strategies recommended by others, and not willing to assume that fibromyalgia was a psychological condition. Thanks to my cranial-sacral and osteopathic physiotherapist, who immediately saw how environmental medicine and the reading group approach supported her work. Without her work, my back might still be 'stuck.' Thanks to my traditional physiotherapist who tried to stop the bull with everything he could throw at it.

A special thank you to a friend who gave me a copy of Betty Macdonald's *The Plague and I*, a book about her experiences in a TB sanatorium for two years back in the 1940s, which affirmed that it is possible to write a humorous book about the most unhumorous subject. Besides this book, there

were a host of others I read in search of understanding of my pain, its causes and possible cures, books by Abram Hoffer, Andrew Weil, Sherry Rogers, Majid Ali, Doris Rapp, Barry Sears, Jeffrey Bland, Peter D'Adamo, Udo Erasmus, Alan Gaby, and others. Because they undertook the arduous and risky task of setting down the results of their experience and experiment, I could access their wisdom over and over as new and confusing issues arose. No doctor, no therapist, however committed, could afford to spend the time that was required to sort out the mass of symptoms. The books gave me many tools and much hope. 'Reading To Heal' became my slogan and the rallying point for the reading groups I formed and the title for another book I have written as a guide to the best information on health and nutrition.

Friends, fellow-sufferers, and reading partners meant a lot. When I became discouraged with some therapy, they would cheer me up and suggest new paths to explore.

And then there is my family, somehow both behind the front lines and there with me in 'no man's land'. For ten years, they have witnessed, coped with, rejected, learned about, hoped, despaired, doubted, and puzzled over my strange battle. Most of all my husband, but my sons and step-mom, too. They have eaten unfamiliar foods, not begrudged the money I spent on vitamins and minerals, listened to innumerable discussions of diet and environmental problems, learned along with me, and shouldered my responsibilities when I couldn't. My sister even grew organic foods for me.

So a big, deep, wide, tall, and strong thank you to Chris, Michael, Matthew, Madge, Barb, Judy, Joan, Mary Grace, Jill, Elizabeth, Ruth, Rose, Lyle, Miriam, David and Kathleen, the members of the reading group such as Marion, Marg, Brenda, Joanne, Jean, and all the others who assisted in this endeavor. Thanks to Bob and Susan for keeping on with publishing the book.

QUARRY HEALTH BOOKS

Fundamentals of Naturopathic Medicine
Dr Fraser Smith
$89.95 CDA/$59.95 USA

Naturopathic First Aid
Dr Karen Barnes
$12.95 CDA/$9.95 USA

The Botanical Pharmacy:
The Pharmacology of 47 Common Herbs
Heather Boon and Michael Smith
$59.95 CDA/$39.95 USA

Maternal Naturopathic Care:
Women's Naturopathic Medicine
Dr Lisa Doran
$49.95 CDA/$32.95 USA

Once A Moon:
From Ibuprofen to Naturopathy
Candis Graham
$19.95 CDA/$14.95 USA

Reading to Heal:
A Reading Group Strategy for Better Health
Diane Dawber
$10.95 CDA/$6.95 USA

Dr Hoffer's ABC of Natural Nutrition for Children
Dr Abram Hoffer
$19.95 CDA/$14.95 USA